INSIDE THE
MAYO CLINIC

Alan E. Nourse

INSIDE THE MAYO CLINIC

McGraw-Hill Book Company

New York   St. Louis   San Francisco
Düsseldorf   Mexico   Toronto

1234567890FGRFGR78321098

Library of Congress Cataloging in Publication Data

Nourse, Alan Edward.
Inside the Mayo Clinic
1. Mayo Clinic, Rochester, Minn.   2. Hospital
care—Minnesota—Rochester.   I. Title.
RA982.R56M46   362.1′1′09776155   79-11285
ISBN 0-07-047493-1

Book design by Roberta Rezk

For GINNY and ROBERT

"We were reared in medicine as a farm boy is reared in farming, and together we began this adventure in medicine, which now seems to be bearing fruit."

—William James Mayo, M.D.
Rochester, Minnesota

1861–1939

Author's Note

It has always been the inflexible policy of the Mayo Clinic that the confidence of its patients be guarded scrupulously at all times and that no patient of the Clinic should ever be identified in any way in the public press or in professional literature. Accordingly, the patient stories recorded in this book, although based on real experiences of actual patients, have been rendered totally unidentifiable in order to protect the privacy and confidence of the persons concerned.

Similarly, it was the request of the Mayo Clinic that no Clinic doctors, administrators or other personnel be mentioned by their actual names. Thus all present-day persons connected with the Mayo institution have been given fictitious names.

The above does not by any means imply any lack of cooperation on the part of the Mayo organization as I gathered material for this book. Indeed, I received most generous and invaluable assistance from innumerable physicians and other personnel of the Mayo Clinic, Rochester Methodist Hospital and St. Mary's Hospital as the book was in progress. Without such support the writing of the book would have been difficult if not impossible, and I am deeply grateful to all these people.

North Bend, Washington   Alan E. Nourse

Prologue

Rochester, Minnesota / *December 1978*

"Let me show you something," the young man said. "You've never seen anything like it in your life, and we've never worked on anything like it before, either."

My host was leading me down a long corridor in the old Medical Sciences Building of the Mayo Clinic complex—an ancient and dog-eared building by comparison to the shiny new Mayo towers on all sides of it. Presently he came to a huge door and threw it open for me. "Take a look at that," he said.

The room beyond the door was built like a huge circular dome, its twenty-foot ceiling laced with I-beams and joists. Light glared down from banks of ceiling spots on the army of workmen laboring below. As for the floor of the place, it looked like the Mayo Clinic equivalent of an unmade bed. Boxes, packing crates and cartons were scattered from one end of the room to the other. Inch-thick insulated cables snaked across the floor. Some of the cartons, partly torn open, revealed very solid-looking chunks of gleaming metal, snarls of colored wires, protruding bolts and rods.

"So what is it?" I asked.

"Just a pile of parts, so far," the young man said. "They're coming in all the time now, and our researchers are doing double time just checking out inventory lists and revising blueprints for getting it all assembled. When it's all together, one part of it will be a three-ton wheel nine feet in diameter. Another part will be a twenty-foot tunnel weighing fifteen tons. Still another part will be one of the most fantastic integrated computer systems ever devised by man." He gestured proudly at the heaps of junk on the floor. "It's our Dynamic Spacial Reconstructor," he said.

"It sounds like something out of 'Star Trek,'" I said. "Just what, exactly, is it going to reconstruct?"

"Human beings," the young man said. "The *insides* of human beings. In living motion and three dimensions and ultimately in color. To be more precise, this machine will provide doctors with a clear, moving, three-dimensional X-ray image of any part of the interior of the human body they might want to see. It will show them any organ they might choose, life-size and in motion, as if the rest of the body weren't even there. The heart, the lungs, the arteries in the brain, the kidneys—you name it."

He told me, then, about the Dynamic Spacial Reconstructor, which could indeed have come straight from "Star Trek" but hadn't. Essentially, the completed device would be an immense and incredibly capable computerized X-ray machine—but an X-ray machine with a revolutionary difference. With this device the patient would be placed on a radio-translucent platform and wheeled into a tunnel in the wall *inside* the machine. The X ray itself would carry twenty-eight rapid-firing X-ray "guns" built into a huge rotating wheel that would revolve around the patient's entire body. Each "firing" of each X-ray "gun" would generate a cone-shaped X-ray image of a portion of the patient's body from a certain angle. As the wheel revolved, each individual "gun" would "fire" swiftly and repeatedly, literally hundreds of times; in the course of just five seconds—the space of about six heartbeats—the twenty-eight units could gather *75,000 separate images* of the patient's entire body, from bald spot to toenails, taken from every conceivable angle, without exposing him to any more dangerous radiation than an ordinary lung scan for cancer.

Then the computer would get to work, perhaps an even more fantastic operation than the X-ray unit itself. Each of those 75,000 sectional images would be broken up into tiny "cubes" of light, as if the entire patient were being minced with a pair of Chinese cleavers. The image "cubes" would then be fed numerically into a superfast computer. Out the other end would come a life-sized three-dimensional hologram of the interior of the patient's body, which could be examined from any angle, studied, manipulated or stored for later reference, whatever the doctors required. Images of individual organs could be separated out and electronically cut open so their interiors could be examined. "There's just no end to the potential uses for this thing," my host declared. "Once it's finished, it could revolutionize the diagnosis of human illness. It could also revolutionize the *treatment* of human illness. Can you just imagine the possibilities if a doctor could actually watch the results of his treatment right while it's going on? Think for a minute and you'll begin to see what I mean."

"I'm beginning to see, all right," I said. "And Mayo Clinic doctors are building this thing?"

"Well, lots of our medical people from radiology and anatomy and cardiology are into it up to their ears. But our major researchers on this project are solid-state physicists, physiologists, biophysicists, computer scientists, electronics engineers, even an applied mathematician. Once they get it all operational, *that's* when the docs will move in."

"And what about the cost of this monster? Or is that a trade secret?"

"No secret. We just don't know ourselves, yet. This one prototype machine already has five and a half million dollars poured into it from the National Institutes of Health and the Air Force and NASA and the American Heart Association. How's that for bedfellows? Total cost may go to fifteen million, but most of that is developmental money. Once it's built and operational and proves itself, most really big medical centers should be able to have one. It'll be too important for them not to."

We poked on around the huge circular room as a crew of workmen demolished another enormous packing case. "So when is this thing going to be on-line?" I asked my host.

"The assembly and installation are already getting started," the young man said. "Then there'll be several months of testing and adjustments, and then a couple of years of animal studies, intensive testing of radiation, meticulous checkout of any possible damage the thing might do. After that there'll be several more years of clinical trials with patients. That phase could start as early as 1982— assuming everything goes right, of course."

"You think maybe it won't?" I said.

The young man scratched his head thoughtfully. "Well, to be perfectly frank, at this point nobody really knows whether this thing is actually going to work *at all* or not. There's never been anything like it before. But then, here at Mayo, we usually manage to get things to work. It's an old, old tradition."

1

Galena, Illinois / *July 1854*

On a hot afternoon in July 1854 two men stood at the rail of the spanking new paddlewheel steamboat as it cast off from the dock at Galena, Illinois, and slipped out into the muddy Mississippi current, heading north toward the Minnesota Territory. One man, tall and hawk-nosed, wore the uniform of a colonel in the cavalry; the other looked like any of a million prosperous young businessmen of the day.

As the shoreline receded, the colonel turned to his companion. "You may be right, Phillips," he said. "With St. Paul growing the way it is, it could be a good place for your branch office."

"I think so," Phillips said. "If my missus can ever manage to make it there." He glanced uneasily back toward the row of first-class cabins. "She's been sick ever since we left Chicago and getting worse every day."

"It's the bad night air," the colonel said. "No good for a delicate creature like her. You should keep those portholes closed at night." He glanced up. "I say, here's an odd-looking chap."

Another man had joined them at the rail, a man so small he barely came up to the colonel's collar. He was young, perhaps in his mid-thirties, with a full black beard, a black frock coat and a black beaver hat that seemed to perch squarely on his ears. Most striking of all were his eyes: deep-set, bright, sharp, observant. When he fixed those eyes on the colonel, the tall Army man found it hard to look away.

They introduced themselves. "A doctor, are you?" the colonel said. "And where are you traveling from?"

"Lafayette, Indiana," the doctor said.

"Indeed! And where bound?"

"Minnesota Territory. I'm not sure where."

"That's quite a jump for a doctoring man," the colonel said. He laughed. "Practice a little slim back there in Indiana?"

The doctor looked up as if measuring the man. "Nothing slim about *my* practice," he said sharply. "It was the fever that got me. Wabash Valley's full of it. Chills and fever week after week, year after year. I finally had enough, so I saddled my horse one day and told my wife, Louise, I was heading west and north till I found a place to practice without any fever, and that's what I'm doin'."

"You mean you just left her there all by herself?"

"She's pretty spry."

The colonel scratched his chin. "Well, you'd better realize that St. Paul is already full of doctors. They don't need any more."

"That's all right. I'll find a place down from the city, maybe in Wisconsin, maybe across the river in Minnesota Territory."

"That's bitter cold country in the winter," young Phillips broke in. "And the summers are too short to grow anything. That means not many people stay around."

"I'll get along," the little doctor said.

"It's also Indian country," the colonel added. "The Sioux are still pretty surly."

"I doubt a few redskins are going to bother me much," the doctor said stubbornly. "I'll just sew them up along with the rest. Now if you gentlemen will excuse me—"

He was turning to go when Phillips touched his elbow. "Doctor, could I have a word? My wife, Liza, is sick, down in our cabin. She hasn't taken nourishment since we left Chicago. If you could just look in?"

"Certainly. Show me the cabin."

Down in the darkened stateroom a young woman was reclining on the lower bunk. The air was stale, the patient almost invisible in the gloom. Phillips introduced the doctor. "Maybe he can help you feel better," he said.

"Might open that port a bit," the doctor said. "Get a little light in here." He pulled up a chair to the bunk and looked at the woman. "You've been sick for days," he said gently. "Now tell me how, and when it began, and all about it."

He listened intently as the woman described her illness. Presently he took her pulse, felt her forehead, listened to her heart and lungs through his wooden-tube stethoscope. Finally he asked the husband for a glass of water and took a paper-wrapped powder from his small black bag. He mixed it and had the woman drink it. Then, with a sigh, he leaned back, took her hand in his and fixed her with an intense gaze. "Madam," he said, "your problem is a traveler's malaise, plain and simple, and I think it will go away now. I think you'll feel well enough this very evening to sip a little broth and take a few steps on the deck before retiring. In fact, I'm sure of it." He smiled at her then, gave Phillips an encouraging nod and took his leave.

Hours later Phillips and the colonel met again at the railing. "Well, our little 'doctor' seems to have retired," the colonel said. "Doctor, indeed! Walking out on a thriving practice, abandoning his wife in Indiana and going off on a fool's errand like this! Believe me, the man's a blackguard through and through."

"I'm not so sure," Phillips said thoughtfully.

"Well, of course, you saw him doctoring." The colonel guffawed. "I trust you stayed close by while he was at it."

"As a matter of fact, I did."

"And your wife?"

"Let me tell you, sir, it was the next thing to miraculous what that man did. He examined my wife and prepared a powder and then looked straight at her and told her she was going to be well. And an hour later she was taking some soup, and just now she paced the deck for half an hour, and she looks like a new woman. And I don't think that powder had a thing to do with it, either. If I didn't know better, I'd say that man works magic."

"Well, magic or no magic, he's still a blackguard," the colonel said gruffly. "*He* won't last long out in the Territory. If the wolves don't get him—or his patients—the redskins will."

"I'm not so sure," Phillips repeated. "He may just do all right, wherever he ends up. In fact, you might be hearing that little man's name far and wide around this country before he gets through." The young man rubbed his chin and stared out at the fading light on the river. "Dr. William W.—what did he say his name was? Major? Mayor? *Mayo?*"

2

Rochester, Minnesota / *April 1979*

The name was Mayo, as everyone living within a 700-mile radius of southern Minnesota today well knows, not to mention most of the rest of the people in the United States and quite a number in over fifty foreign countries as well. The name of that odd little doctor on the riverboat is especially familiar to the people of Rochester, Minnesota, a town of some 60,000 people stuck out in the cornfields a couple of hours' drive south of Minneapolis. In Rochester, without much trouble, you can find a Mayo Clinic, a Mayo Building, a Mayo Medical School, a Mayo Graduate School of Medicine, a Mayo Medical Student Center, a Mayo School of Health Related Sciences, a Mayo Foundation for Medical Education and Research, a Mayo Clinic Board of Governors, a Mayo Foundation Board of Trustees, a Mayo Foundation House, a Mayo Memorial Park, a Mayo Civic Auditorium, a Mayo Medical Museum, a Mayo Senior High School and, somewhere off in the rolling woodlands to the south of town, a stately mansion known as Mayowood. In Rochester, Minnesota, you fairly trip over the name of Mayo, whichever way you turn.

To say that Dr. William Worrall Mayo "did all right" when he settled in the Minnesota Territory in the 1850s is like saying that the Pacific Ocean has a bit of water in it. The little doctor from Indiana, joined by his wife in the new country he had chosen, ultimately found his way to the little crossroads village of Rochester. There, with the aid of two thoroughly remarkable sons and a number of other brilliant people, he proceeded to build the groundwork for a medical establishment of a sort the country had never before seen or even imagined.

Today that establishment has become one of the largest, most prestigious and powerfully influential private medical institutions in America. The Mayo Clinic staff today numbers some 688 fully qualified physicians, including specialists trained in virtually every medical and surgical specialty known to man. In addition, another 680 doctors-in-training are working at the Clinic or in adjacent hospitals, ranging from the greenest intern out of medical school to the fifth-year specialty Fellow* about to qualify as a full-fledged specialist himself. There are also some 10,000 or more other personnel associated with the Mayo Clinic and its affiliated hospitals—multitudes of nurses, receptionists, laboratory and X-ray technicians, other technologists, clerks and office workers, right down to the ever-obliging blue-clad young men stationed at the entrances to the Clinic, and here and there about the lobby, to make themselves useful to Clinic patients in any reasonable way possible.

Even knowing this, it is still a little staggering to learn that a total of 275,000 patients are treated at the Mayo Clinic each year and that since the present record-keeping system was established in 1907 more than 3,370,000 separate patients have registered at the Clinic, with many, of course, seen over and over by Clinic doctors throughout the years. But the power and influence of the place is even more pervasive than such figures would suggest. Young doctors completing part or all of their specialty training at Mayo's have carried the Mayo prestige with them wherever they went in their medical careers. These onetime Mayo trainees have spread out far and wide throughout the country and world. Indeed, by latest estimate, 2 percent of all specialty trained physicians practicing in the United States today have taken part or all of their training at Mayo's. One doctor friend of

* The Mayo term for doctor-in-training or resident physician.

mine trained there in his specialty in the 1950s before moving on to the South to practice; subsequently his younger daughter, after completing medical school, went back to Mayo's for *her* graduate medical training and is now practicing in California, perpetuating the Mayo mystique there in her own quiet way.

Quite aside from treating an ever-increasing multitude of patients each year and training droves of young physicians who later spread all over the country to practice, the Mayo organization has a third strength that places it in the top rank of American medicine: the sheer volume of high-quality medical research that is carried on there, year in and year out. Any doctor on the Clinic staff may, if he wishes, undertake research projects, with all the facilities he might conceivably need located within a couple of blocks' walk. Some of this research is clinical—working with patients, studying the diagnosis, treatment and evaluation of disease. Some is "pure" or basic research, seeking the breakthroughs in scientific knowledge on which tomorrow's new medical advances will be based. Some Mayo researchers spend full time in their laboratories; others divide their time between patient care and research. In any event, Mayo scientists are constantly reporting their work at medical meetings all over the world, publishing their findings in the professional journals in a steady stream, and a great many Mayo doctors are widely known by name and highly respected throughout the world of medicine.

It is no mean organization, this house of medicine for which William Worrall Mayo built the groundwork more than one hundred years ago. It seems ridiculous, in a way, that this huge and multifaceted medical center should be located in a small southern Minnesota town through which you can easily walk in less than an hour. Even today Rochester is obscure and oddly difficult to get to. No passenger train comes to this town any more; the days of the special Joseph Lister coach from Chicago with doors wide enough at the side to admit a stretcher are gone forever. If you go to the bus station in St. Paul or Minneapolis and get on the right bus, you will eventually arrive in Rochester. By car, if you look hard enough, you can find a four-lane highway, Route 52, leading south from the Twin Cities to Rochester, but it is poorly marked and extremely difficult to find. (Curiously, this road becomes two-lane immediately *beyond* Rochester.) The town can also be reached by Route 63 and Interstate 90 from the south.

Far more important for access today is the small but modern airport south of the town which handles a total of forty-six incoming and outgoing flights per day. These flights originate from as far afield as Kansas City, Denver, Miami, Dallas, St. Louis and Washington, D.C., as well as from Chicago and New York. One airline serving the Twin Cities from both coasts makes no additional charge for a round-trip dogleg diversion to Rochester and back from Twin Cities Airport. Despite such air service, there are still a great many people who just can't believe that Mayo can be where it is; every day people disembark from airplanes in Rochester, *New York*, and try to get a taxi to the Mayo Clinic. Airline clerks there have learned from long experience just to tell these people to get back on the airplane and go west to Minnesota.

Certainly the most startling approach to the town is by road from the north. The Minnesota countryside is fertile, rolling farmland, beautiful if a little monotonous, with patches of woods interspersed with hills and homesteads. In the winter, before the snow comes, it looks cold and forbidding, a land of browns and grays and blacks, solid unadorned earth colors. By May green leaves appear in stark contrast to the rich black of newly plowed fields. By August these fields are verdant with soybeans and endless miles of twelve-foot-high field corn, dazzling green and tasseled. As you drive down through this country you are constantly reminded of the mixed historical heritage—agricultural and aboriginal Indian—in the place names you encounter: Shakopee, Wanamingo, Red Wing, Farmington, New Market, Cannon Falls, Blooming Prairie, Mantorville, Zumbrota and Mazeppa. And then, just as you think you *must* have gone past Rochester without noticing, the road ascends, and there before your eyes, rising unbelievably out of the soybean patches, is the Emerald City of Oz!

Not emerald, perhaps, but certainly a city. Skyscrapers! In particular, a tall, solid monolith of gray-and-white marble rising from the center of town, surrounded by a complex of lesser buildings on all sides. The road signs say ROCHESTER NEXT 2 EXITS, but you would be hard put *not* going into Rochester at that point. The road builders assumed, with perfect logic, that anyone who has come that far wants to.

Once off the highway, you are in the center of town in approximately two minutes. Dominating everything is the nineteen-story Mayo Building itself, surrounded by smaller buildings of the Mayo Clinic Complex and the huge Rochester Methodist Hospital. But by this time you are thinking of hotels, not clinics. All the way down the road you've been assailed by billboards for hotels and motels, large, small or indifferent, all suggesting a wildly festive air (swimming pools, deluxe suites, gourmet dining), as if you were arriving for a honeymoon in the Catskills. No truth to those billboards, of course. For one insane moment you imagine them as they might be: COME DIE WITH US AT MCBURNEY'S—CROHN'S INN, RECOVER FROM BOWEL SURGERY HERE!!—MOTEL GRANULOMA, SOFTER BEDS TO SUFFER ON—but no. From the billboards you'd think you had reached the resort capital of the entire Midwest. But *all* the ads do emphasize one true thing: *how far they are located from the Clinic.* "Easy walk to Mayo's," one will say. "Just across the street from the Clinic" or "Fall out your window and you're there."

And in fact, next to the Clinic Complex itself, the hotels are the single most striking thing about Rochester. The town is crawling with them. Directly across the street from the Mayo Building is the large and prestigious eleven-story Kahler Hotel, a rambling edifice with shopping arcades on both ground and basement floors, a genteel lobby filled with overstuffed furniture reminiscent of the 1930s, an enormous dining room with white linen and crystal chandeliers and waiters tiptoeing by on inch-thick carpet. The Kahler sports a roof-garden café with a splendid view of the only thing in Rochester there is to view—namely, the Mayo Building—and a number of the slowest elevators west of the Susquehanna River. "Modest" accommodations here begin at $35 or so, double occupancy, but you can easily spend $65 or $70 a day if you want to—up to $225 a day for suites!—and some of the hotel's services are fascinating if not downright bizarre. Where else in the *world* can a hotel guest dial the hotel Service Officer for an enema and be told "Certainly, Madam, the nurse will be up in just a few moments"?

Other hotels cluster in a ring around the Clinic Complex—the Zumbro, the Hotel Arthur and the Heritage House, among them. Smaller, less pretentious places are available a block or two away: the Clinic View Motel, with undercover parking, at $28 a day, for example, or the Carlton Manor for $18. Farther away is a sixteen-story Holiday Inn, complete with adjacent parking garage, and the Soldier's Field Motel. Both provide free limousine service to and from the Clinic. At still greater distances are smaller, less expensive motels, including a Motel Six out on the highway.

In all, the town's thirteen hotels and thirty-one motels provide some 3,500 first-class rooms for visitors, all within easy access to the medical facilities. But even more striking is the wide variety and availability of tourist rooms in private homes—that venerable American travel institution from the 1920s and 1930s, now virtually extinct everywhere else in the country. A multitude of homes in Rochester display discreet placards in their windows: GUESTS WELCOME; PRIVATE BATH; KITCHEN PRIVILEGES. These relics of a bygone era are still very much alive and well today in Rochester, Minnesota. Some five hundred such rooms are available.

As to the rest of the city, it looks very much like any of thousands of other medium-sized towns throughout America, except possibly duller. Although the Clinic is, in every realistic sense, the "center of town," the main downtown shopping area lies two or three blocks to the east. Aside from a striking superfluity of drugstores, this stretch of town is like something straight out of *Main Street:* a couple of small and overpriced clothing stores, a stationery store, two or three liquor stores, a scattering of lawyers' and dentists' and architects' offices, a small but handsome public library, an occasional grocery store and a couple of movie theaters. There is even a pornographic bookstore, looking just as shabby as such establishments always look, with its windows blanked out with orange paint and a hand-lettered sign on the door announcing hours of business.

A short drive south from the center of town will take you past a beautiful and expansive park on the banks of the Zumbro River, crowded with people picnicking on the grass in the shade of huge spreading trees during summertime, deserted and desolate-looking in the winter. Still farther along is a crossroads shopping center and an enormous shopping mall, well removed from the city center, including a vast supermarket, dozens of service establishments, a large liquor store with the most incredible selection of imported wines you might ever have laid eyes on, a J. C. Penney's, a Sears and a large and handsome new branch of Dayton's Department Store. This suburban-type shopping center is matched by two others, also on the periphery of town but one to the north and one to the west. Among them they provide a touch of modern civilization that seems almost jarring in this small city.

By contrast, a brief walk through the residential sections of Rochester, especially through the older parts to the west and south, gives you the distinct impression that you've somehow been whisked by time machine back to a sleepy little Midwestern town of the 1920s. Block after block of homes are typical: modest residences of white clapboard, sometimes with age-darkened brick or stone trim; front porches with gables supported by stone pillars; two-story edifices with many-valleyed roofs, asphalt shingles and neatly painted downspouts; houses with deep bay windows looking out on front or side yards or, sometimes, built into hexagonal two-story towers at the corners of the building; houses with vast, grassy front and back yards shaded by ancient elms, maples, oaks or sycamores; street numbers tacked to the lintels of the doors or over the porches; and uneven sidewalks, often aging and cracked, providing the walkways from block to block. Nowhere to be seen are such things as the row houses and high-rise apartments so common to the East or the apartments around inner courts so beloved of Californians; they've never quite reached Rochester, Minnesota.

In this part of the city St. Mary's Hospital, a long mile from the Mayo Clinic Complex, fits in perfectly, a rambling brick-and-stone building two blocks long which shows every evidence of having been built—as indeed it was—a piece at a time over the years. Except for the cluster of motels, small hotels and tourist rooms nearby, the hospital could easily pass, at first glance, for a slightly dilapidated college dormitory or the home office of an old and rather seedy insurance company. To the south behind the hospital the ground rises to a sort of hill—the only real hill in town—with its streets lined with somewhat larger homes and dominated by an imposing structure of red brick, complete with its odd-looking four-story observatory tower, once the home of Dr. Will Mayo and his family, now devoted to the teaching activities and medical meetings of the Mayo Foundation.

Still farther west and south on the far side of the hill the homes become more modern: small ranch-style houses, brick-faced, with attached garages, driveways, small yards and children playing on tricycles under the shade trees. And where in this city of doctors are the splendid doctors' homes? The handsome palaces? The grand estates of the princes of Rochester's major industry? Don't look, because you won't find them. You will search in vain for a Beverly Hills of Rochester, and it may strike you that something here is very odd. If you look closely you may see an occasional Porsche, Mercedes-Benz or Jaguar sitting in the driveway of one of these modest-looking homes, but for each one of those you will see a dozen battered Ford station wagons, five-year-old Chevys or Dodge pickup trucks.

It is to the center of activity in Rochester, the Clinic Complex itself—the "Mayo Campus," as they like to call it—that you must go to find the polish and glitter and modernity of the town, and even here you will find curious discrepancies. The dominating structure of the Complex—in fact, the single dominating landmark in the entire city—is the Mayo Building itself, an immense four-wing building rising a sheer nineteen stories from the ground without setbacks, faced in beautiful panels of light- and dark-gray Georgian marble. Here the entrances lead into an enormous lobby, spacious and well lighted, two stories high, which might seem an extravagance until you consider that more than 1,000 people at a time can be, and often are, seated in that lobby waiting for their initial Clinic appointments, surely the largest doctors' waiting room in the world. At one place in the lobby there are wheelchairs stacked, row upon row, like shopping carts in a supermarket. At the curb outside is a thirty-second parking zone to speed up the traffic in taxis, limousines, private autos and hotel vans unloading patients—but the rule is never enforced if it takes a little old lady more than thirty seconds to clamber out of her car. At one place in the lobby banks of telephones line the wall, all busily occupied much of the time. Nearby you will find ranks of stamp machines beside a post box with hourly pickup—and where else but inside a U.S. Post Office can you put 25¢ into a stamp machine and get 25¢ worth of stamps out? At Mayo you can.

It is in this main-floor lobby that the hundreds of patients streaming into the Clinic each working day of the year are greeted at the reception desks. Elsewhere in the lobby are the business desks where patients receive their bills and make payment arrangements before they stream out again. The seventeen floors above the lobby house laboratories, administrative offices, examining rooms and the multitudes of offices where the doctors see the patients.

The time is long past, however, when all major activities of the Mayo Clinic were confined beneath one roof. The Clinic Complex today is made up of a total of eight or more buildings, depending on how you count them. Second largest, after the Mayo Building, and directly across 2nd Avenue S.W. from it, is the fourteen-plus-story Plummer Building, named for Dr. Henry Plummer, one of the earliest and most brilliant members of the Mayo Partnership. This building was the main Mayo Clinic building until the construction of the new marble giant across the street. It is made of tan-colored brick, with arched windows and balconies visible on the upper stories, rococo trim around the top and gargoyles guarding the high-rising carillon tower with its pyramid roof.

In all respects the building stands in quaintly old-fashioned contrast to the sleek modern lines of the new building. The lobby is large and dark, lined with heavy wood-and-leather furniture. Today the doctors' offices are gone, replaced with clinical testing laboratories, treatment areas, administrative offices, medical library and other aids-to-function, all crammed into space along narrow, dark corridors and serviced by elevators that work best (and none of the best at that) when someone is there to hand-operate them.

The Plummer Building also contains the Board Room for the use of the Mayo Foundation Board of Trustees in years past, its walls encrusted with framed citations, awards, diplomas and honorary degrees received by the two Mayo brothers during their lifetimes. Here also are the Mayo archives: glass cases filled with pictures and documents, others filled with the academic robes and hoods worn by the Mayos at ceremonial occasions during the years of their ascendancy. Finally, preserved as a museum, are the only doctors' offices left in the building—the actual offices used by Dr. Will Mayo and Dr. Charlie Mayo themselves at the time of their deaths in 1939 and kept essentially unchanged, as well as the office used by Dr. Charles Horace (Chuck) Mayo, son of Dr. Charlie, until his death in 1965.

If the Plummer Building seems a musty symbol of a bygone era, the Conrad N. Hilton Building for Laboratory Medicine and Center for Research—latest of the buildings to be dedicated—is precisely the opposite. Connected to the Mayo Building by way of a long, bright subway corridor, the main reception room for patients is underground but lighted by skylights and decorated by gardens and plantings. More than anything else it looks like a set from a science-fiction movie. It is here, at the infamous Desk C, that patients present themselves to yield up blood, urine and other samples of bodily fluids for laboratory examination or to receive instructions for other more complex laboratory studies too grisly to mention. Most of the laboratory work is actually done on the floors above, while other parts of the building are devoted to research in human behavior. Above ground the outside of the building, four stories high, sports clean, modernistic lines, stucco facings and tinted glass windows. Completed in 1974, the place was built with a gift of $10 million to the Mayo Foundation from Conrad N. Hilton. Superstrong foundations were provided to support far more weight than necessary, and fixtures on the roof are in place to adapt additional stories in the future when they become necessary. Nobody seems to doubt that that time will come.

Another gift, some $8.5 million from the Murry and Leonie Guggenheim Foundation, was used to meet about half the cost of an immediately adjacent building devoted to research and education in the life sciences. The Guggenheim Building, on 3rd Avenue S.W., a block south of the Mayo Building, is a ten-story structure faced with a highly reflective copper-colored material. The first two floors are used by the new Mayo Medical School, which had its beginning on September 7, 1972. The rest is devoted to other aspects of medical education and research. The building houses lecture rooms, laboratories and demonstration theaters for undergraduate and graduate medical students.

In addition, a Medical Sciences Building of earlier vintage is still standing and still used for research laboratories. Certain floors of this building, reeking of formalin, house the Tissue Registry—hundreds of thousands of preserved pathological specimens removed from Mayo Clinic patients at surgery, all neatly labeled and kept in little glass bottles on row after row of shelves so that (at least theoretically) anyone interested in examining a certain individual gall bladder removed by Dr. Will Mayo in 1912 could do so. Like the Plummer Building, the Medical Sciences Building shows its age and its era and reminds you once again of the steady growth of this institution since its beginnings well before the turn of the century, expanding a step at a time as the work to be done here has increased. Even more striking in this respect is the so-called 14 Building, a small six-story building of aged red brick huddling next to the Plummer Building. This was the first single-building headquarters for the Mayo

Clinic, used by Will and Charlie Mayo and their growing group of associates between 1900 and 1914 for offices and laboratories. Now empty and condemned, identified only by a brass plaque on the outside wall, the 14 Building today is doomed to the wrecking ball.

Three other more modern features of the Complex each have their own peculiar individuality. One is the Curie Pavilion for Cancer Research and Treatment. All that can be seen of this building is an odd little circular glass gazebo standing in a grassy, parklike area to the north across the street from the Mayo Building. This structure has a door but contains nothing inside but a circular staircase and an elevator, both leading downward. The rest of the Curie Pavilion is underground and houses the treatment and research facilities for one of the largest and most active cancer centers in the world. Long underground corridors lead to the cobalt, X-ray and other radiation therapy facilities, special laboratories and treatment rooms for chemotherapy, banks of computers for cancer researchers to use in their work and multitudes of offices and conference rooms. The ground above is occupied by—of all things—a four-story parking garage in the so-called Damon Building, which also provides space for a small medical museum.

Another building is perhaps oddest of all: the Harwick Building, a seven-story lump of concrete, almost totally without windows, a building into which no one, it would seem, is ever seen going in or coming out. It is the only building in the Complex where patients ordinarily are *never* seen, for it is here that are stored the records of the 3,370,000-odd patients who have registered at the Mayo Clinic since the numbering system was instituted in the early 1900s. Another floor of the Harwick Building is devoted to a staff cafeteria; still others house computers used by the Mayo organization, as well as the Department of Medical Statistics so vital to most medical research today. In 1979 a new addition to the Harwick Building was under way, and just southwest of it the newest building of the Mayo Complex was opened: a Community Medicine Building built specifically to meet the medical needs of the Rochester community, as opposed to the rest of the world combined.

One final curiosity of the modern Mayo Clinic plant, and surprisingly vital to the smooth functioning of the place, is the intricate system of subway walkways and tunnels that interconnect the buildings of the Mayo Complex, with branches to the Kahler and Zumbro hotels and to Rochester Methodist Hospital. Branching from a large arcade under the lobby of the Mayo Building, where an extensive newsstand and a large branch of the Webber and Judd drugstore are located, these tunnels reach each of the other buildings and provide access by staircases or elevators. Additional tunnels are used primarily by Clinic personnel—clerks, nurses, receptionists, administrators, engineers and doctors—to get from Point A to Point B with surprising rapidity. On a sunny spring day this system of subways, some one and one half miles of underground walkway in all, might seem superfluous—but midsummer in Rochester, Minnesota, can be hellishly hot above ground and winter can be ungodly cold. For sick patients, for whom the Clinic primarily exists, the subways, built in the 1930s, have proven a remarkable boon.

Not precisely a part of the Clinic Complex but very closely associated is the modernistic Rochester Methodist Hospital, just across the grassy park from the Curie Pavilion. Like other buildings in the vicinity, the Methodist Hospital has grown a chunk at a time, originating with the old Colonial Hospital built by the Kahler family in the early 1900s, soon after it became clear that a hospital closer to the Mayo Clinic was going to be needed in addition to St. Mary's Hospital a mile away. The Methodist Hospital purchased the Colonial Hospital and remodeled it in 1953; in 1964 construction was started on a new hospital just west of the Colonial, a block north of the Mayo Clinic, with dedication in October 1966.

Since then two separate additions have been built, leading to a total hospital capacity of 990 beds. (St. Mary's and Rochester Methodist between them now provide close to

2,000 hospital beds and soon will be providing more.) In building later portions of the hospital, many experimental innovations were attempted—cantilevered sun decks, "pod" type nursing units and a variety of other configurations of patients' beds and nurses' stations, all built in search of the ideal.

But the strangest part of the whole hospital is the now disused and condemned upper-story portion of the old Colonial Hospital, still standing like a corpse that hasn't yet fallen over. Here, through special fire doors, you can travel five feet and step from the most modern of hospital facilities of 1979 into the narrow corridors and antiquated operating rooms of a hospital of 1917. Dust lies thick on the floor; plaster is cracking on the walls and ceiling. What once were patients' rooms are now crammed with dusty, stained, rusty, disused and obsolete equipment—ancient scrub sinks, antiquated plumbing equipment, broken-down operating tables, instruments and carts and stacks of moth-eaten linens, lab benches and glassware, the refuse from an earlier age of medicine, discarded and stored with typical Midwestern frugality for some possible later use that never came and still sitting there in a kind of homely splendor today. Here, I think, more than anywhere else in Rochester, I was struck with an overwhelming sense of the immediacy of history; you could hear world-famous footsteps echo in these corridors. Here we stood in the very operating rooms that the Mayo brothers themselves had used in the halcyon days of their growing fame: tiny, cramped little rooms with white tiled walls and bathroom-tile floors; operating tables still in place, filling most of the floor space; two-tier visitors' galleries for observing surgeons, guarded only by chrome-plated bars and so close above the scene of battle that the observers were literally breathing down the necks of the surgeons; old-fashioned surgical lamps hanging askew on their swivels from the ceiling; tiny windowless, airless rooms in which a major part of the real history of developing American surgery was made.

The impact was incredible. These men and other brilliant ones were *here* in these tiny rooms. One day, no doubt soon, these cubicles will be demolished, along with other older rooms and buildings from the history of the Mayo establishment—but I wish someone would first stop and think about it. I could not help but feel that if ever an authentic museum of a past age of American medicine were to be preserved anywhere, this would be the building in which to preserve it.

This, then, is the modern Mayo Clinic in its external shell, "skyscrapers growing out of a soybean patch," as one administrator described it. But who are the doctors who work here, and what do they do that is different from doctors anywhere else? Who are these 275,000 patients who come here each year? Why do they come in such numbers and from so far away? To find answers to such questions we must go back for a moment to the feisty, bright-eyed little doctor on the riverboat 125 years ago and the remarkable medical dynasty he founded in southern Minnesota with the strength of his own determination and the aid of those two quite remarkable sons.

3

LeSueur, Minnesota / *1854–1863*

Dr. William Worrall Mayo did not establish his medical practice in Rochester when he first arrived in the Minnesota Territory in 1854. Rather, he settled near the small town of LeSueur, some ninety miles west and north of Rochester on the banks of the Minnesota River. There he bought a small farm and sent for his wife and a small daughter who had been born during his wanderings.

The LeSueur area was true wilderness country in the 1850s, abutting on the land of the Minnesota Sioux Indians, a people with whom a very uneasy truce was maintained by means of Indian Agency hand-outs. It was a land where rivers were crossed on rickety ferries, a land through which prairie schooners rumbled, twenty or more a day, on their way to the supposedly more favorable Dakota country to the west.

Even LeSueur was not remote enough to satisfy the little doctor's wanderlust. Hardly was his family settled there than he was off by himself for a look at St. Paul. There he found too many people and far, far too many doctors to suit his liking, so he headed up the St. Croix River to Duluth, a tiny wilderness outpost at that time, and from there, by canoe, up the north shore of Lake Superior, first only as far as Knife River but then farther and farther north, exploring. Ostensibly he was paid by a mining company to inspect copper claims in this remote area, but the main truth was that he was looking to see what he could see and loving it.

Finally he returned to LeSueur and the long-suffering Mrs. Mayo and settled down more or less seriously to practicing medicine. In those days, however, this did not mean precisely what it means today. There was nothing that even remotely resembled a hospital anywhere near LeSueur, Minnesota, and nobody would have gone near it if there had been. Indeed, nobody in those days called a doctor at all unless someone in the family was *in extremis*. People suspected—with canny good sense—that most doctors of the time had little if anything more to offer than they themselves did. No one would think of calling a doctor to attend the delivery of a child unless mother or baby or both were clearly in desperate trouble. Maternal mortality in childbirth was frightfully high, but probably no higher than if a doctor had been on hand. Child mortality was staggering; no one would dream of assuming that any given child was going to survive its early years once it was born, and scarcely a family existed that had not lost at least one child in infancy, if not two or three or more. Even the Mayo's own first-born child, a son, had died at the age of six months, and later they lost a daughter shortly after her first birthday. As for adults, the picture was scarcely better. Death at an early age from infectious diseases was commonplace. Comparatively few survived long enough to become vulnerable to cancer or heart disease in middle age, and high blood pressure wasn't even recognized to exist.

This state of affairs was not the fault of the doctors. Their training was universally poor because there wasn't any good training to be had and very little valid medicine to be learned. True, doctors became familiar with a few ancient and effective drugs: digitalis from the foxglove leaf for heart failure; quinine for the "shaking chills"—the malaria that drove Dr. Mayo out of Indiana; colchicine for gout; and a few others. But beyond this there was little that doctors could offer in treating medical illnesses. And as for surgery, at least in the wilderness areas, this was confined almost totally to lancing boils and amputating gangrenous limbs. Without a safe, effective anesthetic there were few kinds of surgery anyone would submit to unless driven to it; a man's hand caught and mangled in farm machinery, a hand that would today be meticulously repaired and might ultimately be restored to use, in those days would almost surely fall victim first to gangrene and then to amputation.

Thus the frontier physician was not particularly busy and certainly not rich. Dr. Mayo had little use for a consulting room, since he generally went to the patient when he was called, traveling by horse and buggy when the roads were passable, by horse alone when they weren't or by sled in the winter. There was a ferryboat that ran sporadically across the Minnesota River; this sometimes enabled him to get to farm homes on the other side. But his practice could not be described as thriving. Not only were patients few, but nobody had any money to pay a doctor's fee. When we see the verdant fields of southern Minnesota today, it is hard to believe how harsh a country it was in those days. The long, bitter winters either froze people out or left them vulnerable to endless bouts of respiratory infection; the hot dry summers baked their crops. Very often if the doctor brought home a half peck of potatoes as a fee for a twenty-five-mile round-trip call on a patient, he considered himself lucky.

In fact, if he had not been an enterprising soul, his own family might well have starved out. Fortunately he was both vigorous and imaginative, and he didn't mind turning his hand to other things when the practice got slow. In those early years in LeSueur, among other things, he engaged in farming, raising eight head of cattle; he practiced veterinary medicine when called upon, quite as happy to treat horses as people if the horses needed the treatment; he served as the local Justice of Peace; he ran the ferryboat back and forth across the Minnesota River, collecting what he could for passage; for a while he ran a steamboat up and down the river—a venture that led to acquaintance and lifelong friendship with Jim Hill, of later railroad fame; he helped to establish and operate a local newspaper for a while; and he got himself deeply involved in local politics.

Last, but by no means least, with the aid and cooperation

of the good Mrs. Mayo, he fathered a son born in LeSueur on June 29, 1861. The boy was named William James Mayo after his father and his father's brother. And unknown to the doctor at the time, the great dynasty of medical Mayos in southern Minnesota had had its beginning.

Certain events that occurred soon thereafter substantially altered the pattern of the doctor's future. For one thing, the Civil War had begun, and in 1863 President Lincoln signed a national conscription act. Dr. Mayo was appointed as one of the examining physicians charged with determining which of the southern Minnesota conscriptees should be taken for service and which would be rejected. It happened that Rochester was the base for this activity for the district, so Dr. Mayo went to Rochester to live for a period of some eighteen months, leaving his wife and family home in LeSueur.

It was a difficult task to fulfill under any circumstances, since nobody wanted to be chosen, and the doctor was strict and abrasive in detecting frauds. Presently he found himself in trouble. During off-duty hours he saw patients privately, and some irritated souls began accusing him of accepting fees to let certain conscriptees off the hook. There is no sound evidence that he actually did any such thing and considerable reason, considering his known character, to think that he didn't. He was presently officially exonerated—but in any case he was far too irritable and outspoken a man to fit well into a sensitive public-service position. Ultimately he was suspended from his post and returned to LeSueur under something of a cloud—but not before he had developed a fondness for the town of Rochester.

The other crucial event happened a bit earlier and was considerably more scary. For some years previously the relations between whites in the Minnesota River Valley and the Minnesota Sioux Indians had been uneasy at best. The Indians were kept more or less subdued by annual payments in foodstuffs and cash from the national government. But in the spring of 1862 the government Indian Agency found it convenient, for some reason, to be several weeks overdue with the cash annuities the Indians were expecting, while also withholding their food (which was already on hand in warehouses) until the Indians had the money to buy it with. This arrangement did not please the Sioux, who were half starved from a long winter and found that local credit was not available to them to buy the food with. A few confrontations, marked by insults from certain of the whites, finally triggered a small-scale but entirely serious Indian uprising against the frontier villages in mid-August. First a lonely farm was attacked, with five white people killed. Then the Redwood Agency was attacked, the traders shot and the warehouses plundered. Next a number of farms around the village of New Ulm were hit.

In the tradition of the American frontier, night riders spread the word swiftly to towns farther down the river. Their response was in the same tradition: A ragtag army of 125 "frontier guards," including three doctors, headed out from LeSueur in buggies, on horseback or on foot to help defend New Ulm. Two rode a buggy with medical and surgical supplies, but Dr. Mayo managed on foot. The siege of New Ulm was no joke. Two people had already been killed and half a dozen houses burned by the time the defenders arrived. Two days later, after a pitched battle, ten whites were killed and over fifty wounded, with numerous buildings on the periphery of the town burned. Busy treating the battle casualties, Dr. Mayo distinguished himself during the fracas not only for his medical ministrations but for his vigorous encouragement of the guardsmen to stand fast against the attackers. Ultimately the Indians withdrew, and the doctor returned home to his wife and three children—but not without his booty: the body of Cut Nose, a giant Sioux brave whom he had once previously faced down in a dispute over a horse on the way to a call at a lonely farm. After carting Cut Nose's body to LeSueur, Dr. Mayo dissected it with typical curiosity. Later the skeleton was cleaned and prepared for display. According to popular mythology, it is still to be seen in the archives of the Mayo Clinic. (There is indeed a skeleton on display there, but no one today is willing to take an oath that it is actually the mortal remains of Cut Nose.)

Whether the little doctor's experience in the Sioux outbreak cooled his enthusiasm for life in LeSueur to the breaking point or whether he merely had come to like the town of Rochester excessively well when he was there as medical examiner, by January 1864 he had decided that he wanted to move east to the larger town. He bought a pair of lots there, built a small house on one of them and moved his family in. The cottage he built was almost exactly on the spot where the first Mayo Clinic building was built more than fifty years later, a fact commemorated on that building's wall by a small metal plaque. And it was in that house, on July 19, 1865, that a second son was born to William and Louise Mayo. This boy was named Charles Horace, since Charles was a family name of the doctor's and Horace the name of their first-born child who had died years earlier. The doctor also built a small office on downtown 3rd Street and notified the 3,000 residents of Rochester of his presence by a small and discreet newspaper ad, brief but emphatic:

DR. MAYO
Office on 3rd Street
Rochester, Minn.

The Mayos were established in Rochester.

4

Rochester, Minnesota / *June 1979*

The patient arrived at Rochester Airport at 5:00 P.M. on a Monday evening on connecting Northwest flight 453 from Chicago after departing from the hospital in Mexico City on American Airlines flight 104 nine hours earlier. She was a thin, wraithlike nine-year-old girl who had seemed three-quarters dead before she ever got on the airplane and didn't look any better now. Two men from the waiting ambulance were at her side with resuscitation equipment almost the moment the plane touched down; another gently took her parents aside—a worried, graying Mexican businessman and his darkly beautiful wife—to assure them they would have separate transportation to St. Mary's Hospital, while others moved the stretcher off the plane and into the emergency vehicle. Then, with siren howling, it was a quick trip for the girl into downtown Rochester and out 2nd Avenue S.W. to the hospital, accomplished in record time; the people of Rochester are used to the flashing ambulance lights along that route and know enough to get out of the road. Within thirty minutes after the plane landed, the girl was in the cardiac intensive-care unit on the fourth floor of St. Mary's Hospital, with Dr. Howard Norgaard, the cardiac surgeon in charge of her care, at her bedside along with a retinue of some eight other doctors, nurses and technologists.

A critical decision had to be made and made swiftly: whether to risk the time necessary to stabilize the child's condition, relieve some of her heart failure, get rid of edema fluid, oxygenate her blood and perform the cardiac catheterizations and the X-ray studies Dr. Norgaard really needed to determine the exact situation with her faulty heart valves before he operated—all procedures which would increase the odds of her surviving the forthcoming surgery if she lived long enough to have it—or whether to forget the studies and take her to surgery then and there in a feverish attempt to rescue her from imminent death. The girl, whom we will call Manuela La Barca, was a child born with multiple heart defects, including a sizable hole in the muscular wall separating the right and left ventricles (the large pumping chambers of the heart) and two imperfect heart valves. One, the aortic valve, was slightly displaced so that part of the blood pumped by the left ventricle went in the wrong direction, throwing an intolerable load on the heart; the other, the pulmonic valve directing blood to the lungs for air, was malformed so that only a tiny stream of blood could pass through, leaving Manuela's body constantly and disastrously starved for oxygen.

The hole in Manuela's heart muscle had been surgically corrected by skilled surgeons in Mexico City when she was a tiny baby. In addition, those surgeons had repositioned her aortic valve to the location where it belonged—but following the surgery that valve had scarred and twisted partially closed. Thereafter the surgeons had replaced both the aortic and pulmonic valves with artificial valves that looked for all the world like pingpong balls in little four-prong wire cages.

For several years Manuela did reasonably well. But unfortunately, as she grew larger, the artificial valves did not. Two years after the first valve surgery, they had to be replaced. Two years later they had to be replaced again—but this time the scarring of tissue around the valves had become so extreme that neither of the new valves fit or worked properly. For three years she limped along, growing thin and weak, short of breath, essentially a crippled child for whom little could be done.

Then, at the age of nine, Manuela's overtaxed heart suddenly began to fail. Examinations showed that the edge of one of the valves had come loose, and the Mexican doctors suspected the other might be weakening. Manuela's illness swiftly advanced from serious to critical. It was then, after a long telephone consultation between Dr. Umberto Garcia-Lopez of Mexico City, one of the finest cardiac surgeons south of the border, and Dr. Howard Norgaard at the Mayo Clinic, that the decision was made to bring the child to Rochester in hopes of salvaging a virtually impossible situation.

By the time Dr. Norgaard reached the cardiac intensive-care unit at St. Mary's, a whole sequence of life-support measures had already been set up by his Chief Surgical Fellow—a cardiac surgeon-in-training with five years' experience—working as a team with a pediatric Fellow and Dr. Charles Hornby, one of Mayo's sharpest pediatric cardiologists, whom Dr. Norgaard had called for help and advice. In many ways the intensive-care unit looked more like a bad science-fiction movie than a hospital nursing unit; it was shaped like a long rectangle lined by a dozen or more patient cubicles, each glass-walled and in full view of the central nursing station. In the station was an electrocardiograph monitor for each patient, plus continuing monitor read-outs for pulse, respiration and blood pressure. In one small room at the side, primarily an X-ray reading room for the doctors' use, there was a monitor read-out screen and two columns of buttons so that the monitoring system for any given patient could be flashed on the screen and checked as of that moment merely by pushing a button.

As for the patient, Manuela already had an intravenous infusion running into her spindly arm; all monitors were functioning; blood and urine samples had gone off to the laboratory for "fastest possible" reports; and initial observations of her arrival condition had already been charted in the standard 8- × 10-inch Mayo Clinic patient file just opened for her, complete with her individual seven-digit case number. Dr. Hornby was just completing a careful physical examination when Dr. Norgaard came in. When he finished his exam, the two men went down to the X-ray reading room to review an initial chest X-ray and check the electrocardiogram together.

Hornby studied the cardiogram at some length, then sighed. "Well," he said, "I guess it's not as bad as it could be."

"Yeah," Norgaard said sourly. "She's still alive."

"On the other hand, she's an absolutely impossible candidate for emergency open-heart surgery."

"I know that, too. The question is, what happens if we *don't* move? Is she just going to go out on us?"

"She very well could," Hornby said. "But there's a hint or two that she may be stabilizing a little. Of course, she's not bumping around in that airplane any more, and that's a help. But she just doesn't look all that absolutely bad to me, right at this moment. I'd like to see her blood studies and chemistries, at least, before you guys start work on her. Be sure she's not in renal failure or liver failure or acidosis or something. I'd also like to get some of this fluid off and get the heart failure under better control before you guys take over."

The surgeon shrugged. "Right now, you're the boss. I don't want to operate on a corpse if I can help it. How much time do you think you'll need?"

"No more than a couple of hours if things start going sour. Maybe until morning or longer if they go better."

"You think we could at least cath her in the morning, then?"

"If she doesn't force your hand sooner."

"Good. Then we'll schedule that for seven, tentatively, and take it from there. Meanwhile, if you think we'd better move during the night, pass the word. No sense taking chances at this late stage of the game."

The tall, lean surgeon went on to make rounds on several other patients in the house, with two of his surgical Fellows in tow. Never the most placid man in the world, Howard Norgaard felt extraordinarily nervous about this new young patient from Mexico. Over the years, in some indefinable way, he had developed a set of deep-seated instincts about patients to which he paid far more attention, in some inner recess of his mind, than he would ever have dreamed of admitting publicly. It was almost as though he could look at a patient from the door of the room, just the briefest of glances, and know in the back of his mind, "This one is going to be all right," or "This one is a bummer." His instinct about Manuela La Barca was not good, and he knew it, and he didn't like it. He wasn't even sure what made him feel this way; he had pulled some awful chestnuts out of the fire in the past, some of them far sicker than this girl—but here, somehow, something was warning him.

He went to a phone, checked with the Clinic to see if the angiograms and other films that had come up with the girl had been brought in from the plane yet. When he learned that they had, he asked that a Clinic shuttle driver bring them over in the van on his next trip. Actually they were already on their way, so he went down to meet the shuttle on the first floor, took the bundle of films back up to the intensive-care unit and began going through them one by one, a long, dismal visual record of operations and failures on the growing girl over the years. The most recent films he studied especially long and intently. *Bad. A bad scene altogether.*

Presently he drove the few blocks to his home, confident that the beeper box he carried on his belt would warn him if he were needed. He leafed through several journal reprints that his wife had left stacked for him on the hall table before she left for her evening League of Women Voters meeting, found nothing very interesting and tossed them aside. He had two other cases scheduled for the next day, but neither one presented any great difficulty. By 10:30 he was about to turn in but decided on impulse to make a final trip to the hospital, just to be sure.

Manuela looked much the same as before, very much awake and alert, toothpick-thin, her skin a pasty gray in contrast to her large, dark-brown eyes and jet-black hair. As he looked at her he could see her sick enlarged heart thrusting against her breastbone, literally jarring her small body with each heartbeat. He knew from Dr. Garcia that she understood English and spoke it quite well, so he tried talking to her, tried cheering her up, but he might as well have been talking to a post; she just turned her head away. Finally he just smiled, touched her forehead, still far too warm, and gave her hand a gentle squeeze before turning and leaving the cubicle. Outside he saw one of his younger Fellows, a dark-haired young man, coming up the hall. "Dr. Ruiz?"

The young man stopped. "Yes, sir?"

"You speak Spanish, don't you?"

"Sure. But not Mexican Spanish. Tucson Spanish."

"Well, there can't be that much difference." The surgeon paused as a nurse drifted by. Then: "That child is terribly frightened."

"Yes."

"You might even say terrified."

"Yes."

"I wonder—could you talk to her a little? In her own language?"

"I can try," the resident said. "What about?"

"Anything. It doesn't matter. Just something to make her less frightened. Ease her mind a little."

"I can try," Dr. Ruiz said dubiously.

"I wish you would." The surgeon paused, looked closely at the young man. "Listen," he said suddenly. "I don't know why, but I think this child is going to die. I feel it in my bones. Yet sometimes what the patient feels, what the patient believes, can make all the difference. And maybe, just maybe, if this child were not so frightened—"

"I'll do my best," the young doctor said.

After Dr. Norgaard had gone, the young man went into the girl's cubicle, alone with her except for the monitoring nurse. Manuela's eyes were alert, watchful. Not in the least trustful.

"I'm Dr. Ruiz," the young man said in her own language. "I came to see if I can help. Are you comfortable now?"

"*Si.*"

"But frightened."

"*Si.*"

"You've had too many operations."

"*Si.*"

"And they haven't helped."

"No."

"But this time maybe one will. You have a fine doctor—one of the finest in the world. He wants this operation to help. We all do."

For just a moment her eyes softened and she almost smiled. "I know," she said in her soft Spanish. "That's why they brought me to Mayo Clinic."

"Then you think about that. Really believe it—this time the operation will work."

Maybe it helped Manuela, the positive thinking approach; there was no way to tell. But for Dr. Norgaard, on his way home, the power of positive thinking was not helping a bit. All he was hoping was that by morning he might feel different.

Not every patient who goes to the Mayo Clinic meets with the kind of speedy and solicitous reception accorded Manuela La Barca, I soon discovered. "Good heavens, no," Art Amundson told me later. "The ordinary run-of-the-mill patient without any really urgent problem who calls today for a date to go through the Clinic is likely to learn that the next firm Clinic appointment available is in fifty-eight weeks or so. It's been as long as eighteen months in the past. But you have to realize that this girl from Mexico you've heard about is a very special case. One phone call from Umberto Garcia-Lopez down in Mexico City and Howard Norgaard was over there at St. Mary's personally scrubbing down the operating room. For one thing, Dr. Garcia is an old, old friend of the Clinic; he's sent us hundreds of patients. But more important, the child was desperately ill. There wasn't even a day to lose, much less fifty-eight weeks."

Art was not a physician at Mayo, but he was an important and powerful man on the administrative staff at the Clinic just the same. As the Director of Public Relations he was a short, stocky man in his early fifties, with a thick shock of iron-gray hair, a gravelly voice and a face that kept reminding me of Boris Karloff. His office on the eleventh floor of the Mayo Building was small and neat, with clean spare lines and a lack of clutter that seemed characteristic of the place. A large picture window offered a splendid view of—what else?—Rochester, Minnesota.

"But why send her *here?*" I asked him. "They do top-rate open-heart surgery down in Texas. That would have been much closer. So would New Orleans or Miami. Why *here?*"

"There's always been a kind of a Latin American thing here," Art said. "You're going to get tired of hearing this, but a lot of it goes back to the Mayo brothers themselves. Surgeons were constantly coming here to watch their work, to study and learn, and those surgeons included a lot of men from Mexico and Brazil and Venezuela and Colombia and Argentina. Will and Charlie always made them feel at home here, always treated them like gentlemen and equals. This was at a time early in the century when an awful lot of American surgeons looked down their noses at anybody who came from south of the border. The Mayo brothers made a lot of Latin American friends just by being decent—and then in 1917 the two of them made a sort of grand tour of Central and South America, just when they were reaching the height of their fame, and it wasn't just the doctors who greeted them down there; it was the *people* who turned out in droves, and those people remembered. And ever since then Mayo is where those doctors and their successors refer their tough cases, and Mayo is where a lot of Latin American patients come on their own. Lots of people in medicine accused the Mayo brothers of self-advertising, and others claimed they were just a whole lot smarter—you know, cannier—than the rest, but I'm not sure those things were on their minds at all. They were good, and they knew it, but they especially liked to teach. They certainly weren't worried about making money by that time—hell, they couldn't even give away what they already had—but they loved surgery and surgeons, and they loved teaching, and they didn't care where the surgeons came from. So that's how the Latin American connection got started."

"Well, that's fine for Manuela," I said, "but what about other emergency patients? You can't seriously mean that all quarter of a million patients who come here each year, sick or well, have to make appointments fifty-eight weeks in advance."

"Oh, lord no," Amundson said. "That's really just a starting place. A lot of our patients are very sick indeed; they need attention right now, and they get it right now. And that includes a lot of drop-ins, too."

"Drop-ins?"

"Patients we've never seen nor heard of before. Patients who come here without any referral from a doctor. They may just arrive from seven hundred miles away without having made so much as a telephone call. They just walk in the door and say 'Here I am.'" Art chuckled. "Like the old guy that Ben Ogilvy operated on the other morning. He's seventy years old and lives in Oklahoma City. He'd been having gall-bladder attacks for the last seven years, and they didn't go away when some doc down there took his gall bladder out five years ago. Well, one day a couple of weeks ago this old fellow had an especially bad attack, he just couldn't get to sleep, and he decided that that was the last gall-bladder attack he was going to have. So he got into his car at three in the morning and *drove* to Rochester. All by himself. Only stopped to sleep once the whole way."

"So what did you do when he got here?"

"Well, we registered him and screened him, set up a Clinic appointment for the next day, and Ben explored his common bile duct two days later. Found a rock in there the size of an olive. Already now his jaundice is clearing up and he's free of pain, and you might say he was a happy man to leave that stone behind, too. It's not an unusual story, either. In fact, it's almost typical."

"So you screen the patients, then," I said.

"We have to, of course. And we have to hold time open on the appointment schedule to provide for the drop-ins who need help right now. The Mayo brothers could be backed to the wall with their scheduled surgery and they'd still always see drop-ins. It got to be policy, back then: never turn anybody away. And we still try to carry it out, big as we've gotten. We actually keep about forty percent of our appointment time open for acute problems that walk in, including time that falls open each day because of cancellations or no-shows. Of course this leaves the doctors a lot of flexibility in the amount of time they can devote to a given patient, too. They never know how much time a patient is going to require for his initial examination, for example, especially a patient they've never seen before. It may take twenty minutes, or it could conceivably take three hours. And since they work on the 'leave no stone unturned' principle, they simply *won't* be rushed. Sure, there are ways to speed things up if they have to, but not at the cost of a sloppy workup."

"Even so," I said, "you must have some way to pick and choose patients."

"You mean among the drop-ins? For a long time it was sort of a matter of first come, first served, but that didn't help when one person had acute appendicitis and another was here to see about headaches she'd had for the last forty-three years. Finally we settled on what we call a priority examination—a brief doctor's exam to determine who needs full attention right now and who can reasonably wait for how long. When somebody turns up without an appointment, or referral, or any Clinic history, we get them in to see *somebody* that day or the next if we possibly can. It's just a screening exam, maybe only ten or fifteen minutes, and it's not supposed to be diagnostic, just enough to determine how urgent the problem probably is.

"For somebody in real trouble, the screening doctor flags the appointment desk and gets that patient an appointment with somebody appropriate for the next possible time slot—maybe right that same day, if necessary, or maybe the next day, or the next, if it's not really a three-alarm fire. If it's only moderately urgent, the screening doctor can ask the appointment desk for the next appointment time that isn't preempted by somebody else. Then the patient checks in with the desk each morning at eight o'clock and leaves a contact phone number and generally gets worked in within three or four days."

"Suppose it's not even moderately urgent," I said. "Just something that needs attention in the next few months, say."

"Probably, then, the appointment desk will find a firm

appointment time a couple of months ahead, set it up on the books and send the patient home with instructions to come back when the time comes. Or they may give the patient the option of sticking around for a few days, checking in each day in hopes of a cancellation. Or they may tell the patient to go home and they'll call him at the earliest possible time that some appointment turns up. Which it may well do. We have some godawful busy seasons, but we have some slack periods as well."

Amundson stood up and gazed out the window at the western part of the town, so thickly planted with spreading shade trees that hardly any houses or buildings could be seen. "Of course, there are other factors the screening doctors try to consider too. A man may not be so desperately ill, but if his problem is keeping him from working, they're going to try to work him in as soon as possible. If they sense a potential suicide situation, obviously they're going to try to get hold of it fast. If the guy is moving into a new job and wants a checkup because he's feeling lousy, that would be taken into account. And then we have our own interests, too. Lots of the doctors here are involved in research programs of one sort or another. If their research is clinical, that can mean finding a large number of patients who are suffering from the sort of problem that they're trying to study. Of course any such research has to have the informed consent of the patient— nothing's being put over on anybody. But if some drop-in patient looks as if he might fit into an important research program after he's gone through the Clinic, that could well get him an early appointment even if he weren't so desperately sick. Basically our job is treating sick patients, but the fantastic wealth of pathology walking through these doors makes it a researcher's paradise too."

In Roger Barton's case, getting an appointment at the Mayo Clinic was the result of a combination of things. For one thing, Roger was indeed ill—but this was a fairly minor part of the picture. After all, he had been ill virtually all his life and had worn out dozens of doctors who had tried to treat him. More important, perhaps, was that Roger Barton was a very imperative and pushy young man who was not inclined to take no for an answer from a bunch of big-name mucky-muck doctors who were probably quacks anyway. But the main factor was something Roger Barton hadn't even thought of and, indeed, didn't even know enough to think of.

Roger Barton was a man who was used to having things his own way. He had lived his entire thirty-seven years in Mason City, Iowa, a not unhandsome young man, never married, just short of six feet tall, heavier than he ought to have been, with a head of glossy black hair of which he was inordinately vain and for which he paid ridiculous sums to have it frequently and properly tended.

Strictly speaking, Roger didn't have to work at all. His father, killed with his mother in an auto wreck when Roger was five, had made a small fortune operating hardware stores in four Iowa counties and had left Roger well off for life under the guardianship of his maiden Aunt Hattie. Aunt Hattie would have much preferred that Roger *didn't* work, because then she could have kept a closer eye on him. But Roger failed to oblige her. After he finished college, more for amusement than anything else, he had taken a job selling insurance to the surrounding farmers and soon had an agency of his own. It was handy because it allowed him to travel to the surrounding towns and villages, spending an occasional night away from Aunt Hattie and generally meeting people, talking to people or going to bed with people as the opportunity arose.

Roger's Aunt Hattie insisted that she took such doting care of her brother's son because he had been ill ever since he was a boy. Some speculated that Roger might have been ill ever since he was a boy because his Aunt Hattie took such doting care of him. Whatever the cause or effect, there was no question that Roger was ill and had been so for many years. He had been the victim of bronchial asthma for as long as he could remember. The asthma attacks were frequent and often severe, sometimes totally disabling for days at a time. Typically, medicines would help his asthma for a while and then quit working. The house he lived in was outfitted with special air filters, blowers, purifiers, dust-free carpets, dust-free drapes and a million other devices to cut down on allergens, and these had worked for a while but didn't any more. His attacks were far worse in the spring, summer and fall than in winter. And in any event, it seemed that the closer he was to Aunt Hattie, the worse the asthma became. The only way to be free of it was to get out of town. But with his agency, this was hard to do for more than a few days at a time.

Roger had other problems too. Along with the asthma he also had a severe nasal allergy and hay fever that kept his nose plugged up and his eyes red and puffy most of the warm-weather season when pollens were about. In addition, he had recently been noticing other things. He was beginning to have bad reactions to medicines—any medicines. One drug that was supposed to abort asthmatic attacks began to precipitate them instead. Another that previously caused no trouble began to nauseate him for forty-eight hours every time he took it. He noticed, on the rare occasions that he engaged in physical exercise, that his heartbeat became irregular whenever he exerted himself. He began having headaches, so he bought a blood-pressure apparatus and started taking his own blood pressure four or five times a day. He never seemed to find it elevated, but the headaches got worse.

The crowning blow came when Roger terrified a young lady from Higgins Corners, Iowa, in a secluded motel room one night at 3:00 A.M. The girl awoke with a start to find Roger simply *not breathing at all* for two and three minutes at a stretch and then gasping and puffing and snorting like a drowning man trying to catch up—without even awakening. Unwilling to be caught with a corpse on her hands in a Higgins Corners motel room that morning, she quietly packed up and left, and when Roger learned the reason from her over the telephone the next morning, he decided the time had come to do something. He had seen every doctor in Mason City, Iowa, so many times that they all ran and hid when they saw him walking down the street, so this time, he decided, he would see what the hot shots could do. He would go to the Mayo Clinic.

He contacted Mayo's in early June, just as the summer pollen season was cresting. His first connection with them was not promising. Transferred to the appointments secretary, he found the young woman extremely pleasant and apologetic but not at all helpful. "I'm sorry, Mr. Barton, the first appointment I can confirm for you would be on November sixteenth."

"*November sixteenth!* That's insane. I could be dead by November sixteenth. I've got to see a doctor *now.*"

"I see. And you say you have no referring doctor?" Long pause. "I'm afraid this is very difficult, Mr. Barton. Maybe it would be better for you to come in, so we could get you on our priority list in case of cancellations."

"Come in? To *Rochester?* Hell's bells, woman. I live in Mason City and I work for a living. How can I just come in?"

"I know it's a long way to come," the young woman said. "But our schedule is terribly crowded right now. We're only booking strict emergencies."

"This *is* an emergency," Roger said, exasperated. "I can't breathe. My heart's jumping all over the place. I'm starting into the pollen season right now and already my allergies are killing me."

"I see. Well, Mr. Barton, let me have you talk to Dr. DeVore, if you'll hold a moment. He's in our Allergy section. Maybe he can help."

Roger thought sure this would mean a twenty-minute wait on the long-distance line, with him paying the bill, but it was more like thirty seconds when he heard a man's voice. "DeVore here. Is this Mr. Barton? I understand you're having some problems."

Roger told him what he had told the girl, with perhaps a trifle less embellishment. The doctor listened, then said, "I suppose this does get to be quite a bother in the spring and summer."

"That's putting it mildly. I can't work, I can't sleep. I

can't do anything. All summer long I sit home with my head in an air filter and even then I can't breathe."

"I see. And antihistamines don't help much?"

"I can't use antihistamines any more. I'm allergic to them."

There was a long pause. "Uh—you mean they don't seem to do much good any more—is that right?"

"No, that's *not* what I mean," Roger said testily. "I mean I'm *allergic* to them. When I take antihistamines I break out with hives and itching and sneezing and nausea."

"Really?" The doctor paused again, even longer. "Now that's *interesting*," he said at last. "That's very interesting indeed. And a lot of this seems to be a nasal allergy as well as asthma?"

"That's right," Roger said.

"Okay, look." Something had changed in Dr. DeVore's voice. "There's no point having you disabled all summer if we can somehow work out an appointment sooner. Let me start checking, right now, and see what's actually possible. Then I'll have the young lady get back to you, probably in an hour or so."

Dr. DeVore took Roger's telephone number in Mason City and rang off. He sat staring at the wall for several moments, then rang a four-digit number on the Mayo Clinic intercommunication system. "Gerald?" he said. "This is Earl DeVore. Are you still running that study on antihistamine-fast allergics? . . . Good, good. And you're still looking for patients? . . . Splendid. I think I've got a live one for you. I'll be seeing him next week. I'll give you a call." He hung up, then dialed the appointment desk girl again and told her what he wanted.

Three-quarters of an hour later Roger Barton had a call from the young woman in Rochester. "Mr. Barton, I think we have things straightened out. You have an appointment with Dr. Earl DeVore next Tuesday morning. You should expect your complete examination to take from two to three days, possibly more. We'll need to have you check in at the appointment desk in the main lobby of the Mayo Building no later than seven o'clock Tuesday morning, so if you're coming from Mason City you'd better plan to arrive in Rochester Monday afternoon or evening. I'm sending down some information about the Clinic so you'll know what to expect and a list of hotel accommodations. You'll be driving? Then allow plenty of time; there's construction on I-Ninety between Austin and Stewartville."

Everything in Roger Barton's nature urged him to insist on changing the time to Wednesday because of a luncheon date on Tuesday, but for once in his life he kept his mouth shut and just wrote down the appointment on his desk pad. After he hung up he sneezed several times, wiped his eyes and took a couple of deep wheezy breaths. *Well, what the hell,* he thought. *Maybe they'll find something that works up there. At least the guy thought I was an interesting case. That's what he said, a very interesting case. That's a lot more than any of the quacks around here ever thought.*

Wheezing like a leaky bellows, Roger Barton arrived in Rochester about four o'clock the next Monday afternoon. It had taken the firmest of persuasion to convince Aunt Hattie that she should not come along "just to have a checkup," since he was going up there anyway. Having made a hotel reservation by phone, Roger left Aunt Hattie sulking in Mason City, got into his car and headed north for the Minnesota border.

The hotel Roger chose was, of course, the Kahler. He had carefully perused the list of accommodations and instantly concluded that none but the closest to the Clinic—and the most expensive—would do for him. He was shown to a small, quiet, third-story room but immediately found this unsatisfactory: too dark, too small, too noisy, nothing to see but a parking lot outside, etc., etc. He rejected three subsequently offered rooms as well on various grounds (after all, he'd seen the tariff list and *knew* what kinds of rooms were available) and finally, to the manager's relief, agreed to accept a master suite on the tenth floor with a southern exposure and air conditioning, a huge sitting room—bedroom arrangement that also happened to be the most expensive accommodation in the house outside of the Bridal Suite.

That distasteful bit of business taken care of, Roger changed, bathed, dressed, called the bellboy for fresh towels, called the bellboy for ice, called room service for appetizers, called the maid to arrange a drape which had come off one hook at the end, and finally, ignoring his Mayo Clinic instructions requesting that a patient take no alcohol the evening before his examination, had three large, stiff bourbons on the rocks in rapid succession, feeling immensely pleased at himself for having refused to allow those hotel types to push him around.

After his drinks were finished he decided to go out, since the evening was mild and the sun not yet set. First he took a turn around the Mayo Building and other buildings of the Clinic Complex, then walked two or three blocks south to Broadway and looked around the town. The Mayo Building he approved of—*that*, at least, seemed to have a little class—but the business district was dreadfully unimpressive, he decided, compared to the splendor of Mason City, Iowa. Even so he took note of a couple of clothing stores and a restaurant or two before returning to the hotel for dinner.

There he presented himself at the Elizabethan Room, the hotel's "quality" restaurant, without a reservation at the height of the dinner hour and then paced impatiently until the hostess finally found him a table. The first one was out in the middle of the dining room, far too "public" to suit Roger, so he sent the maître d' scurrying until he could find him a table suitable for four in a secluded alcove. He had a couple more double bourbons and then (again ignoring the Mayo Clinic advice to take a light evening meal the night before his exam) proceeded to stuff himself with dilled Swedish salmon, vichyssoise, beef Wellington, two glasses of sherry, a bottle of French burgundy, an enormous salad, a gooey dessert that mounded up on his plate like Mt. Everest, two cups of coffee and three after-dinner brandies.

Back in his room, he checked his blood pressure but found it the usual 120/80. He spent an hour or so perusing one or two of the publications he had purchased at an unsavory bookshop downtown, had two more drinks, called someone to adjust the air conditioning (which he decided was not working properly because his asthma was becoming severe) and ultimately retired for the night.

He didn't sleep too well (he often didn't) but finally dropped off about 2:00 A.M. Since he'd neglected to set a clock or leave a call, it was seven minutes after 7:00 A.M. when he finally came to life. He called room service for a leisurely breakfast, showered while he waited for it to arrive and presently walked in the main entrance of the Mayo Building at ten minutes of eight. Following the directions of a blue-uniformed young man at the door, he found his way to the Admission Section with its main desk at the front and its long line of desks stretching beyond down a room a half block long. Facing these desks, in a waiting section, were row upon row of chairs, some three hundred of them, and virtually every one of them was occupied. He presented his appointment card to a pleasant-looking middle-aged woman at the main desk. She nodded, glanced at the clock and asked him if he'd mind taking a seat until his name was called. He sat down and waited some forty minutes as patient after patient was called to one or another of the desks. Finally, as he was considering walking out, he heard his name called, directing him to desk No. 7.

"I say," he said to the young girl in the cubicle, "I happen to be a rather sick man. Is all this waiting entirely necessary?"

"I'm sorry, Mr. Barton, but we had to reschedule your appointment with Dr. DeVore this morning, and now we're waiting for a possible opening. We asked you to be here at seven, and we had you scheduled for his first appointment, but I'm afraid it's far too late for that." She handed him a small light-brown paper wallet with a white stripe across the top bearing the letters E-14, stamped with Roger's name, his address, Dr. DeVore's name and a number of letters and numbers that he couldn't decipher. "If you'll take this up to the fourteenth floor, east side, and give it to the girl at the desk there, she'll get you to see Dr. DeVore as soon as possible—surely *some* time today."

There was some small delay while Roger, inattentive as ever, found his way to West-13 by mistake, stood in line waiting to hand the appointment wallet to the girl at the desk and then had to be redirected to East-14, but he finally got there. The receptionist handed him a lengthy folded questionnaire, a writing board and a pen and asked him to fill out the form and return it to her as soon as possible. Once again, he was startled at the sea of seats in the E-14 waiting room, two hundred or more, most of them filled. It occurred to him that if this single half of one floor of the Mayo Building was any example, a great many people were sitting in waiting rooms in this building waiting to see doctors. He sat down and filled out the questionnaire (except, of course, for those questions he regarded as "none of their business") and returned it to the girl at the desk. She said she would call him as soon as Dr. DeVore could see him.

As it turned out, Dr. DeVore couldn't see him for quite some time. Patients were called one by one and escorted by attractive girls in white uniforms down corridors to the left or right of the reception desk; patients emerged and departed for other places; new patients came in, stopped at the front desk and then took seats. Not all the patients were pleased; not all were even pleasant. Some complained bitterly about one thing or another; some wanted to see a doctor other than the doctor they were assigned to; some complained about delays; one matronly lady complained loudly and bitterly that she'd been put off for four days straight when all she wanted was to see Dr. Tomlinson for ten minutes; and through it all the girls at the reception desk were the epitome of diplomacy and quiet helpfulness. They were pleasant, they were sympathetic, they were unflappable. What was more, in a simple and orderly sort of fashion, they seemed to get things done.

Clearly these women were persons in authority, empowered to fill the time of the doctors on E-14 as judiciously, economically and usefully as possible. Roger had assumed that Dr. DeVore would have an office, an examining room, a receptionist, a couple of seats in his waiting room, and that would be that. In point of fact, there were a dozen different doctors' names listed on the small call board posted near the reception desk for this single half-floor of the Mayo Building, and these three women were constructing the schedules for *all* of them as people came and went or as time appeared or vanished.

For lack of anything better to do as he waited, Roger studied the personnel. Two of the women at the reception desk were in their mid-thirties, while one was perhaps fifty. The older one greeted all incoming patients and handled most queries while the other two worked around her. One seemed primarily in charge of opening a tubelike gadget and taking out plastic-covered folders that measured about eight by ten inches; another was mainly occupied filling out appointment slips and assembling cards which went into patients' appointment wallets. The folders went into an odd mechanism that seemed to be a continuous moving belt that disappeared through the wall behind the reception desk, each folder going into an upright slot. Both these two were also constantly on the telephone. All were efficiently attractive—*but hardly my type,* Roger reflected.

The other personnel were the escorts who appeared at either end of the desk, picked up microphones cradled there and announced the names of patients they were ready for. These girls, mostly blond and blue-eyed, were much younger, perhaps in their late teens or early twenties. There seemed to be four or five of them who worked in tandem, and they gave the distinct impression that they were moving *fast.* Indeed, none of these women seemed to be sitting around drinking coffee. And if there was something disturbingly robotlike about this operation, well, at least it got things done. Certainly this brass-tube affair was robotlike—*whisk* and *thunk* and out came another plastic-covered folder—and then there was this never-ending belt that went clickety, clickety, click out of the hole in the wall at one end of the reception desk and back into a hole in the wall at the other end, carrying those plastic-covered folders in its gentle metal teeth. Robotlike? Surely not the women—but awfully efficient for humans just the same.

Roger Barton waited for an hour, an hour and a half, his patience wearing thinner by the moment. Other patients came and went, and still he sat. He was just deciding that ten minutes more and he was going to get out of there, doctor or no doctor, when he heard his name called by an absolutely stunning young escort girl. Unfortunately, as she approached, he saw that she was wearing an absolutely stunning engagement ring with a wedding ring tucked behind it. *Ah, well, can't win 'em all,* he thought. The girl led him down a corridor and into a small empty room. She gave him a devastating smile. "Just have a seat in here, Mr. Barton, and Dr. DeVore will be with you in a few moments," she said.

The room was perhaps ten feet by twelve, and it was the oddest doctor's examining room Roger had ever seen in his life. At one end, above a three-foot ventilator, was a tinted plate-glass window looking out to the east of town. Along the right-hand wall was the doctor's desk and chair; next to it was a small Danish modern sofa, lean, spare and comfortable, for the patient. Across the room was an examining table, with blood-pressure apparatus and eye and ear instruments plugged into the wall on spiral cords—and that was all. At first Roger couldn't pinpoint what, exactly, seemed so strange; then he realized it was the very *bareness* of the room. There were one or two nondescript pictures on the wall opposite the sofa, a couple of magazines in a rack next to the sofa and nothing else. The doctor's desk was perfectly bare. Even the top of the ventilator, normally the perfect catch-all for papers, books and other paraphernalia, was built at a 45-degree angle so that anything placed on it would simply slide off onto the floor.

Roger sat down to wait, and this time the wait was brief. Within five minutes a young man in a conservative business suit came in and introduced himself as Dr. DeVore. "Sorry to hold you up so long," he said with a sigh. "This day has turned into a real dog."

"Is this kind of wait normal?" Roger said.

"A little too normal these days," DeVore said. "We're three men short in this section right now. One's on vacation, one is down in Miami at an allergy meeting I was hoping to go to, and one just left the Clinic to become the Chief of Allergic Diseases at the University of Kansas Medical Center. So those of us here at home are running ourselves ragged."

The doctor leaned back in his chair and looked at Roger. DeVore couldn't have been more than thirty years old, an unimpressive little man with a bland, affable face and blond hair, balding a little. "I went over the history sheet you filled out a little while ago," he said, "and there are a few things there we need to double-check."

With that, Dr. DeVore began double-checking every single item on the history sheet. This time Roger chose to answer the questions he had neglected to answer before. The doctor probed the history of his allergy and his asthma as far back as Roger could remember. Indeed, he went into exhaustive detail about the nature of these illnesses, when and how they occurred, things that seemed to trigger them—every item of information imaginable. If he had complained of being rushed off his feet before, he showed no sign of being rushed now. Frequently he would pause for as much as half a minute at a time, scratching his chin and looking at the wall. He checked on Roger's medication history and found a recurrent pattern: any medicine that Roger had ever started he had invariably discontinued almost before it could have had any effect at all. This seemed to fascinate the doctor. "Why did you quit all these medicines?" he asked.

"They just didn't agree with me," Roger said.

"You mean *not one* of them agreed with you?"

"Not one."

"Well, what exactly do you mean when you say they didn't agree with you?"

"If it wasn't one thing, it was another," Roger said. "One pill would make me feel like throwing up all day. Another would make me itch. Another would give me headaches. Another would make my heart jump."

"And not one of them had any effect on the asthma?"

"Well, maybe a little. But then the help would wear off. And somehow the ones that seemed to help the most would always be the ones that disagreed with me the worst, so I had to stop them."

"And this antihistamine thing was the same old story, I suppose."

"Right—excepting worse."

"That's absolutely fascinating," Dr. DeVore said, staring at the wall and musing for a while. Then he went on to check out other things: Roger's gastrointestinal function, his kidney function, his heart function and so forth. Finally he asked Roger to undress down to his shorts and sit on the examining table. The doctor then performed a painstaking physical examination. As he started to take Roger's blood pressure Roger told him: "You won't learn anything from that. It's always normal."

"Oh, really? How do you know?"

"I check it all the time. I've got my own blood-pressure gadget."

"And it's always normal?" The doctor went on checking, took the cuff off and checked it in the other arm. "I wouldn't say it's exactly normal right now."

"You mean it's high?" Roger laughed. "Yeah, I've had other doctors tell me that too. So then I go home and check it and it's perfectly normal. I think I just get hyped up sitting in a doctor's office."

"But we've been doing nothing but sitting here quietly talking for the last half hour," Dr. DeVore protested. "I'm not so sure your blood pressure *is* always normal. Maybe when I see you next you could bring your blood-pressure gadget along and let *me* take your blood pressure with it."

"You can do it right now," Roger said. "I've got it right here in my briefcase." He hauled the pressure cuff out and presented it proudly to Dr. DeVore.

"Show me how you use it," Dr. DeVore said.

Roger put the cuff on his arm and took his blood pressure the way he always did. "There now," he said. "See? One twenty over eighty."

"Good. Now let me try it." Dr. DeVore took the instrument, glanced at it, worked the valve on the rubber bulb a time or two, then puffed up the cuff and fiddled with the valve to try to get it to release the air. The air only went out when he shook it a couple of times and held it upside down. "I'm afraid you've dropped this thing on the floor once or twice too often," he said. "It isn't working."

"You mean I've been getting a bum reading all this time?"

"Could be. But why guess? We can find out what your

blood pressure *really* is doing, under controlled conditions, down in our blood-pressure lab while you're here." DeVore motioned for Roger to get dressed while he went back to sit at his desk. "In fact," he said, "there are a number of things we need to check out in order to get a really thorough look at what's going on with you. First off, of course, we'll want a variety of lab studies, checking your urine and taking blood for a battery of chemistries. Then we need to know how your lungs are really working. The pulmonary function lab is the place to find that out. Don't worry about whether you're having an asthma attack at the time or not; we can take care of that. But among other things we need to know is how much of your trouble is asthma and how much is bronchitis and determine how much underlying lung damage you have, if any. Then I'd like you to see Dr. MacMichael—he's a rhinologist—and find out what he thinks of that badly deviated septum you have; that could be part of your breathing problem at night. I think some allergy testing is in order and perhaps some medication testing as well. Incidentally, you might just possibly be interested in a special allergy study we have going at the present time. Nothing to do with your examination or treatment, but one of our men, Gerald Fried, is working on a new way of treating allergic people who can't use antihistamines. He's following a group of patients who have both asthma and other allergic problems. You might think about seeing him, and we can talk about it later. Meanwhile, you're going to have a couple of busy days."

"You're not going to give me any medicines?" Roger said.

"Not right now. First we need to sort out what's been going on with the medicines you've already been taking and then see if we can pin one down that will really help without causing you trouble. And the blood pressure checking, too; that could be the most important thing of all."

The doctor stood up. "If you take a seat out front, the girl at the desk will call you as soon as she has your appointment folder put together, maybe fifteen or twenty minutes. I'm going to want to see you again day after tomorrow, to brief you on what we've found out."

"Then you do think I have a problem?" Roger said.

"You've been sitting here for over an hour *telling* me you have a problem. Well, I believe you. I also believe that with a little patience and perseverance we can do a whole lot to get rid of it. But a lot will depend on you." Dr. DeVore looked straight at Roger. "With all these various lab appointments and tests, the timing and the instructions are critically important. They may seem silly to you, but they're not. I want you to follow them *to the letter* from now on, like it or not, even if they're a great big bother. It could make the whole difference in how successful we ultimately are."

With that the doctor shook hands with Roger and disappeared back down the corridor as his patient returned to the front desk. Roger sat down and waited as the girl put together his appointments and lab instructions. Glancing at the clock on the wall, he saw that his first encounter with Dr. DeVore had consumed a solid hour and twenty-five minutes.

Mildred Jordan Hulbert, an eighty-year-old grandmother from Denver, Colorado, came to the Mayo Clinic with a different sort of problem and in a completely different sort of way.

Millie Hulbert had been a Minnesota girl almost all her life. She was born and raised in Bemidji, a small town a couple of hundred miles north of the Twin Cities, and knew almost everybody there on a first-name basis. Her own parents and their respective families, large clans of Minnesota people, had been going to the Mayo Clinic since the early 1900s; the place had no mysteries for her. She had married and moved to the East for a dozen years or so, but when her husband met an early death from cancer she had moved back to Bemidji again with its old friends and familiar surroundings.

For years she had taught in the local grade school there, never inclined to remarry. Then came retirement. The old family house was a burden to keep up; one by one her old friends were either passing away or moving to Florida or the Southwest, where the winter weather was kinder. One day Millie woke up and said to herself, "By golly, I'm going to Denver. I've got enough money to manage with. My son and his family live there, so I could be reasonably near them. I'll just find a nice condominium with no house or garden or yard to have to worry about personally. Anyway, I've always wanted to go to Denver."

She moved at the same time that her last old Bemidji friend, Ada Tornstrom, moved to a retirement home down in Minneapolis. Millie liked Denver. She was a bright, alert and active woman despite her age and had a multitude of interests. But every year in early summer, like clockwork, she flew out to Minneapolis to visit Ada for a couple of weeks.

It was on the seventh or eighth such trip, when she was eighty-one, that Millie happened to find a lump in her breast during her shower one morning.

Millie had already had one brush with cancer. Some four or five years before, a mole on her thigh had begun to enlarge. A nice young surgeon in Denver had done a biopsy and then excised the lesion, together with a four-inch margin of tissue all around it. It made quite a hole in her leg, but it healed quickly and didn't bother her much. The surgeon had said the thing was a malignant melanoma and that he thought it was probably eradicated. Even so, he had wanted her to check with him every year, without fail, to be sure there was no recurrence.

She'd regarded that as a trifling matter, but a lump in the breast was something else. And whether he was nice or not, she decided that the young surgeon in Denver was not the person to go to. As far as Millie was concerned, for something potentially serious you went to Mayo Clinic.

She discovered the lump while bathing on a Wednesday morning at Ada's, and as soon as she was dressed she sat down at the telephone. She did not, however, call the Mayo appointment desk. Nor did she ask to speak to someone in the Department of Surgery. Rather, she asked to talk to Dr. Timothy MacMichael, who happened to be an ear-nose-throat man.

It did not strike Millie Hulbert as the least bit irrational to call an ENT specialist about a lump in her breast. She had known Tim MacMichael all her life. As a girl she had known his father, who had also been an ENT man at the Mayo

Clinic. Once or twice she had met his son, who at present was a Fellow in ENT training at the Mayo Clinic. For many years the MacMichaels had had a summer place on Big Turtle Lake north of Bemidji, right next to Ada Tornstrom's cabin and Ada's parents' cabin. In the old days it had been a long hard day's drive for the doctors to get up to the lake place from Rochester, but when the new landing strip was built nearby, Tim could fly up almost every weekend of the summer to join his family and do some fishing.

She had the doctor on the line almost as soon as she had given the receptionist her name. "Tim? This is Millie Hulbert."

"Millie! My dear, it's good to hear your voice! Are you calling all the way from Denver?"

"Heavens, no. I'm here in Minneapolis visiting Ada."

"Ah yes, Ada. I haven't seen Ada since last Thanksgiving."

"I know she was in Rochester then," Millie said, "and that's why I'm calling. I think I may have the same problem Ada did. I found a lump in my breast this morning."

"Oh, dear. I see. Well, of course we know that those things are usually benign—but we really can't take any chances with them." The doctor paused for a moment. "Look, there's a young fellow here named Jerry Whitehead, a very careful young surgeon. I'd like him to have a look at this. Could you come on down here today? I'm sure I can talk him into checking you tomorrow morning."

"Well, Ada could drive me down," Millie said, "but I don't know what the hotel situation is."

"Oh, forget about hotels," MacMichael said. "You can both just stay at the house. Our daughter Jane's up in the Cities taking some summer courses, so we have two guest rooms that are vacant." He thought again for a moment. "Tell you what, you come on down this afternoon and we'll all go out to dinner at the Candlelight. Mary'll be glad for an excuse not to cook. Meanwhile, I'll get things set up for tomorrow."

When Ada came in with the groceries, Millie told her about the turn of events and the plans she had made. "Well, that's fine," Ada said. "When it comes to something like that

I believe in taking the bull by the horns. It's a pretty drive this time of year and I haven't seen Tim in a coon's age. So let's just get a few things packed."

By two in the afternoon they had their "few things" packed and were heading south toward the Mendota Bridge and Highway 52 to Rochester. Millie Hulbert found herself looking forward to seeing Tim and Mary MacMichael again with such pleasure that she almost forgot the unpleasant and threatening reason for going in the first place.

Rochester,
Minnesota / *1865-1880*

Dr. William Worrall Mayo's practice in Rochester during the first few years was a sometime thing. His earlier trouble there as examining surgeon for conscriptees probably didn't help any, nor did his fiercely outspoken and opinionated manner. There was no single public issue of any importance in the entire community about which Dr. Mayo didn't have a firm opinion, and there was no opinion he held that he didn't thrust upon people, loud and clear. True, he made many friends as a result of this, because his opinions were often very sound— but he also made enemies.

Even worse for the practice, times were not good in Rochester in the late 1860s and early 1870s. The great wheat-handling business which had made the town so prosperous a few years before quite suddenly collapsed as the railroads jacked up their shipping fees out of reason and the big-city wheat buyers dropped their purchasing prices. People in the town and on the nearby farms began going bankrupt and moving away. Nobody had any money, least of all to pay doctor bills. One of Dr. Mayo's earliest private patients in Rochester was a sick horse that a local farmer called him out to see. It didn't matter to Dr. Mayo—a patient was a patient, as far as he was concerned—and if his fee was pretty small, his successful treatment of the beast probably helped his local medical reputation more than if he had been treating the farmer's wife. Minnesota farmers in those days had a very direct sense of values.

Very slowly, however, the practice did at last begin to grow. In his spare time, Dr. Mayo got involved up to his ears in Rochester community life. He served on the school board, urging the building of a new school. He tormented the local citizenry into establishing a city library and stocking it with books, many of which he donated from his own shelves, and he helped plan a series of talks by visiting lecturers which he felt certain would help improve the minds of the local farmers. As time went on, the doctor was after people in rapid succession for a city waterworks, a gas works, an electric light plant, a system of sewers and a city park. He was a prickly man to have around.

As for the practice, it was primitive and makeshift at best. Virtually the only medical examining instruments that existed at the time were the clinical thermometer and a crude wooden stethoscope. There was no accurate way to do a complete urinalysis; Mayo did his best by boiling down a bit of urine in a teaspoon to see if it grew cloudy (indicating protein) and testing it for sugar, and that was about it. He did have an ancient low-powered microscope, but it could have been of little use indeed for observing cells in the urine, and the routine blood counts of today were far beyond the technology of the time. For his diagnoses the doctor had to depend, for the most part, on what the patient could tell him and what he could see with his eyes and feel with his hands.

Nor was there much opportunity to compare notes with other doctors in the region. Writing down case records was not yet a common practice, and such few medical histories as were recorded bore little resemblance to the orderly, complete case histories doctors depend on today. In a three-year period from 1866 to 1869, Dr. Mayo kept only about a dozen handwritten case histories dealing, for the most part, with cases that had baffled him. Still and all, he *did* feel the need of contact and discussion with other doctors, and in 1869 he joined with some physicians in St. Paul to breathe new life into the state medical society. He remained active in that organization for twenty years.

When it came to treating patients, this was even more sketchy than diagnosing their problems. The little doctor could lance a boil, set a broken leg and hold it in place with splints, apply hand-made salves and ointments to skin lesions, apply mustard plasters and poultices when he felt they were indicated, sponge down a fever or administer the very few medicines that he knew to be active against one or another illness, but beyond that there was really little he could do. The vast amount of Dr. Mayo's treatment involved the use of an enormous mental storehouse of empirical tricks and trials—the things that he knew sometimes worked, drawn from long years of experience seeing patients and trying somehow to help them. Above all, he relied on the one great medicine that worked better than anything else: *tincture of time*—the knowledge, also drawn from experience, that with sufficient time, rest, support and encouragement the human body can do a remarkable job of healing itself in the vast majority of cases, whether a doctor is there or not.

By the early 1870s the pace of the practice began to increase, although there is no evidence that it brought the Mayo family any but the most modest subsistence-level livelihood. Meanwhile, the boys too were growing. Young Will Mayo was ten or eleven years old, his brother Charlie six, and the two had become an inseparable pair. They were very different people, those boys, even at that age. Will was tall, thin, light-haired, blue-eyed, a loner, neither seeking nor accepting close friendships, stubborn, already a little arrogant but physically strong enough to back it up. Charlie, on the other hand, was short and stocky, brown-eyed, affable, maker of friends and leader in mischief, but tending to be "sickly" according to early records. Different as they were, the friendship between the two brothers was already there and already showing signs of becoming unbreakable. They were a familiar sight together on the streets of Rochester, "those Mayo boys," and all their contemporaries knew that if you picked a fight with one of them, you were going to end up fighting both.

In 1875 Dr. Mayo bought a farm on the outskirts of Rochester, and the family moved out there to live during the summer months. Charlie took to the place and developed a lifelong love of farming; Will did not. Will liked to ride horses, while Charlie preferred to tinker with machinery. When something broke down around the house, he was the one who could always make it go. Mrs. Mayo kept a comfortable home within the means available and devoted her spare time to such interests of her own as botany and amateur astronomy.

All in all, at this point in his life William Worrall Mayo could have taken satisfaction in his growing practice, his own delight in fast horses and his growing influence in local and state politics (in 1890 he was elected to a four-year term in the state senate). But for all of this, Dr. Mayo still was restive.

The trouble was that deep in his heart of hearts the doctor wanted to be a surgeon—and there wasn't any such thing, to speak of, in central Minnesota in the 1870s.

Of course, surgery was done there—when it absolutely had to be. When such a grisly occasion arose, it was like a torture scene from a bad grade-B movie. A farmer, for example, might catch his foot in the belt of a threshing machine and be dragged free with his leg reduced to a mangled hash of torn-up flesh and bone halfway up to the knee. He would be carried, intermittently howling and fainting, into the farmhouse kitchen and laid out on the table. Presently the doctor would arrive, in his muddy boots, well-worn trousers and dusty black coat. Experience told him instantly that the extremity had to be amputated. If it weren't, it would soon become a festering mess; then it would become gangrenous and would very probably kill the victim if pain, shock and blood loss didn't take care of him first. His chances of survival might be slightly—*very* slightly—improved by amputation.

If the patient were conscious, the doctor would order him to be given four or five fingers of potent raw homemade whiskey and would then settle back to wait for it to take effect. Presently the doctor would wash his hands in the kitchen sink (perhaps), dry his hands on the family towel, extract what few surgical instruments he owned either from the bottom of his black bag or from his vest pocket, wipe them on his pants, order the farmer's three hulking sons to hold the man down, and then proceed with the amputation, making it as mercifully short a procedure as he could. Big-name city surgeons of the day built their reputations on the fact that they could do an amputation of the thigh in ten minutes flat. The small country surgeon could not hope to be so swift. He would use turpentine to staunch the blood flow, make as good an attempt as he knew how to close the skin over the amputated stump, step back from the table, wipe his bloody hands on his trousers and restore his instruments, after scraping off the blood and gristle, to the bottom of his bag for the next call of duty.

That accomplished, the country surgeon would sit back to observe his results, none too hopefully. In many cases blood loss, pain and shock would shorten his vigil considerably. If the victim lived, within twenty-four hours he would have a raging fever. In forty-eight hours the stump would be oozing pus. If the patient's natural physical resources and resistance were exceptionally strong, his body would slowly fight off the ravages of infection. Over a period of days the drainage of pus from the wound would gradually abate, perhaps aided by the doctor's opening an area that was "pointing." The terrible pain would gradually, gradually ease. In maybe two months or so the patient would be able to be up and around for a few hours a day on a homemade crutch. Later, perhaps, a son would whittle an artificial foot and ankle out of a piece of cordwood—or he might have the stump fitted with a peg-leg end. Either way, the farmer could count himself exceedingly fortunate to be alive.

That was surgery in the back country of America in the early 1870s, scarcely more than 100 years ago. It was hardly any wonder that nobody cared to submit to it who didn't have to. And aside from amputations, setting of broken bones, lancing of boils and stitching up gaping wounds, that was very nearly the limit of what the back-country doctor could or would attempt in the way of surgery.

The picture was not a great deal different in such sophisticated centers of medical progress as Philadelphia, New York, Boston or Chicago. True, there had been pioneering surgeons who had taken the risk of doing major surgery in America decades before. As early as 1809 a surgeon named Ephram McDowell in the frontier town of Danville, Kentucky, had opened a woman's abdomen to remove a huge ovarian tumor. His attempt was either rash or heroic, depending on how you look at it; according to folklore, his medical colleagues stood outside on a street corner while he was at work, debating whether, when the woman died, McDowell should merely be charged with malpractice or arraigned for manslaughter. Thanks to kind Providence the tumor was safely removed, the woman survived for over thirty years and McDowell's name went down in surgical history. Somewhat later a certain Dr. John Bobbs of Indianapolis placed himself in similar jeopardy by opening a patient's abdomen, incising his gall bladder and removing stones from it.

In another instance, as early as 1840, an Alabama surgeon named James Marion Sims had learned how to do surgical repairs of the vagina. It was he who invented the familiar duck-bill vaginal speculum for vaginal examinations out of a pair of teaspoons and drew silver wire sutures (which he thought led to less infection) out of half-dollar pieces. By the 1860s and 1870s Sims had become quite famous for his new surgical methods for treating gynecologic diseases. Meanwhile, in 1845, two surgeons in Lancaster, Pennsylvania, named John and Washington Atlee improved on the crude method McDowell had used for the removal of his patient's ovarian tumor. By 1870 one of them had done no fewer than three hundred such operations—but a full thirty percent of Atlee's patients had died.

Pain and high mortality rates were the two great obstacles to surgical advancement which seemed insuperable at the time. General anesthesia using ether had first been successfully attempted by Dr. Crawford W. Long of Jefferson, Georgia, in 1842 and was later reintroduced by William Morton, a dentist, in Boston in a famous demonstration in 1846. The doctors there who saw it used were impressed; the patient could quickly be rendered totally unconscious and insensitive to pain. Unfortunately, ether was also a dangerous poison. The dosage had to be skillfully calculated to produce the necessary results, no more and no less. Patients given too little had a way of waking up in the middle of a painful procedure and leaping off the table, while those receiving a bit too much never woke up at all. Chloroform had the same general anesthetic effect but was even more dangerous, with a tendency to destroy liver cells, so the patient who was saved by surgery might later die of liver failure. To top it off, Dr. Long and William Morton engaged in a long and acrimonious battle over who should have credit for introducing ether; for some obscure reason, Long had failed to report his early use of the substance until 1849, when Morton's claim was well established with the profession. This created precisely the kind of malodorous public mess that smacked of quackery and made fashionable and reputation-conscious surgeons reluctant to have anything to do with the anesthetic. It was not until fifteen years later that use of general ether anesthesia became widespread among city surgeons; its use did not filter out into the back-country practices for another ten or fifteen years.

High mortality rates were an even worse problem, and the be-all and end-all of that problem was infection. Surgery and infection seemed to go hand in hand. Virtually every surgical incision, large or small, anywhere in the body, became infected. Indeed, it was a common notion at the time that the formation of a large quantity of pus in a surgical wound was a *good* sign of healing. Doctors even called it "laudable pus." But such infected wounds could also easily develop into blood poisoning or gangrene and lead ultimately to death. To make a surgical opening into a patient's abdomen was to guarantee peritonitis, with a high risk of subsequent death or, at the best, the formation of an internal abscess that could produce prolonged illness. There seemed virtually nothing that anyone could do about this, and it meant that staggering numbers of surgical patients—20 percent, 30 percent, 40 percent or more, depending on the operation—did not survive their surgery.

Oddly enough, two men in Europe in the early 1860s already held within their hands the final answer to this frightful problem and did not even know it. In Paris a young French chemist named Louis Pasteur was busy devising elegant proofs that all infections were caused by *bacteria* — tiny plantlike organisms that covered the body, lived in the earth and traveled in the air. At the same time, a Scottish surgeon named Joseph Lister had slowly come to the conclusion from his observations that the festering wound infections which led to so many tragic deaths were actually produced by something in the air surrounding the patient — but he had no idea what that something was. It was not until 1864 that Lister read of Pasteur's work. A year later, in 1865, he began applying the powerful antiseptic carbolic acid to the gauze used for cleaning his patients' surgical wounds — and found his surgical mortality rate reduced dramatically. By 1870 word of these two men and their remarkable joint discovery had filtered across the Atlantic, but it caught the attention of virtually no one. It would be another ten years — at least — before American surgeons would begin putting the work of Lister and Pasteur to good use and the barrier of surgical infection would crumble beneath a staggering wave of surgical advancement.

In the late 1860s Dr. Mayo of Rochester did not yet know of Pasteur's and Lister's momentous discoveries. But as early as 1866 he had bitten the bullet and made a small abdominal incision in a female patient in order to drain the fluid from a huge ovarian cyst, the first doctor in Rochester to embark upon such an adventure. The operation was written up in the August 25 edition of the Rochester *Post* (as was the custom of the day) and the patient lived. Whether it was this publicity or the nature of things in the area, Mayo soon found himself swamped with patients suffering from a wide variety of disorders euphemistically known as "female problems."

It was hardly surprising that the women in the area suffered such problems sooner or later; they must have had the most overworked female genital organs in all history. These women, for the most part, had married lusty young pioneer farmers. Many were married at age fourteen, fifteen or sixteen and began conceiving children without an instant's delay. To their farmer husbands "many children" meant "prosperous farm," especially when the children were boys who would presently do their share of the hard manual labor of pioneer farming. Those women would have baby after baby after baby, conceiving the next one just as fast as they could after the last one was born. Ten or twelve children in a farm family was hardly worth passing notice. Many women had fifteen. Some had as many as twenty. Birth control was simply and literally unheard of. Prenatal care, by and large, was also unheard of. Babies were born at home with the aid of a midwife (or a husband or daughter) far more often than with the assistance of a doctor.

As might be expected, infection at childbirth was commonplace. So were vaginal and rectal stretching and tearing, lacerations of the cervix, overstretching of the ligaments supporting the uterus and a dozen other conditions related to the trauma of childbirth. Vaginal tearing often led to the formation of vesicle-vaginal fistulas—abnormal openings between the urinary bladder and the interior of the vagina, a condition that left the victim without bladder control, constantly dribbling urine into the vagina, with no hope for control. Women developed ovarian cysts—benign tumors in which a sac of fluid, sometimes as large as a basketball, would form around the ovary. Other women developed cancer of the ovary or the uterus. Most common of all was retrodisplacement of the uterus, a condition in which stretched or damaged supporting ligaments allowed the uterus to tip backward onto the floor of the pelvis rather than tilt forward above the pubis where it belonged, causing the victim all manner of pain and discomfort. Doctors would try to treat this condition by having the woman insert an oblong ring of wood or metal known as a pessary into the vagina in hopes of tilting the uterus forward and holding it in the proper position, a treatment that seldom worked very well and certainly could not have won any popularity contests with the women.

With so many women suffering this kind of pathology, and with the little doctor's growing reputation as one of the best doctors in Rochester, he found himself called upon to treat more and more such "female problems"—but all too often he simply couldn't help because he didn't know the best techniques and had no experience. We can imagine him fuming in frustration, pacing his office floor and muttering to himself, kicking the wastebasket, glaring out the window with those piercing eyes of his, his bearded chin thrust forward defiantly. It was not in his nature to encounter a roadblock like this and not find a way around it—and find a way he did.

He knew that these women could be helped only by surgery. He also knew that certain surgeons in the East were doing such surgery with what was then an "acceptable" mortality rate of only 20 to 30 percent. If William Mayo was going to do such surgery in Rochester, Minnesota, he was going to have to find out how to do it from somebody who knew. Finally, in the fall of 1869, he packed his bags, bid his family goodbye and headed for New York City. There he spent several months studying general surgery and in particular gynecology—the diagnosis and treatment of "female problems"—in the surgeries of the most noted surgeons of the day. Then, before returning home, he traveled to Lancaster, Pennsylvania, to visit John and Washington Atlee, the surgeons who had become famous for performing surgery on ovarian tumors. Most of their operations involved opening the abdomen and draining huge ovarian cysts, but in other cases they had actually removed diseased or cancerous ovaries as well. One of the Atlee brothers had done 300 such operations at the time Dr. Mayo visited, with an average mortality of 30 percent. At the time, this seemed to Dr. Mayo to be a little more radical an operation than he wanted to undertake, with a little too high a mortality rate, but there is no question that his visit with the Atlee brothers fired his enthusiasm for female surgery and made him all the more determined to make this field of medicine his own area of expertise.

Upon returning home, he not only initiated what he had seen the Eastern surgeons doing; he innovated as well. For example, he had observed surgeons doing surgical repairs of cystoceles and rectoceles—conditions in which a portion of bladder or bowel pouches out into the vagina, usually as a result of damage sustained while bearing numerous children. These operations did not involve entering the abdomen and often healed well, but the repairs were not very strong and frequently broke down after a couple of years. In 1871 in Rochester Dr. Mayo attempted a different sort of vaginal repair. Instead of just excising the outpouched bit of organ and then sewing the hole shut as the Eastern surgeons did, he pushed the outpouching back into its proper location and then formed overlapping flaps of external tissue, much like a double-breasted jacket, to provide much stronger support. This proved so successful that he was soon doing vaginal repairs on women from far and wide.

Of course, much of his growing practice was far more routine—seeing babies with the summer colic, treating women with headaches and men with splinters in their thumbs. But the surgery continued, both for "female problems" and other things. He continued to innovate, often departing from customary practices that he thought were bad. He was uneasy, for instance, with the common practice of amputating any injured or wounded limb that seemed likely to get infected and tried to limit his surgical excision to tissue that was obviously diseased, crushed or irreparably injured, doing his best to preserve what appeared healthy or might heal. He reasoned that a farmer with just half a foot would at least be better able to continue his farm work than if he had a stump ending below the knee with a peg attached. His approach drew a great deal of criticism from other doctors in the region, but this didn't bother Dr. Mayo a whit, and he didn't seem to suffer any shortage of patients on account of it.

Ever since the early days of William Mayo's practice people have wondered why the Mayos, in all their growing fame, always chose to remain in Rochester. Why didn't they go to a major population center like Minneapolis or St. Paul? Surely there were more patients there. More opportunities for money and fame. Interestingly enough, early in 1873, when his local fame was beginning to spread, Dr. William Worrall Mayo *did* go to St. Paul for a while to practice. At that time he was serving as president of the state medical society. He was also eager for more surgical experience, and colleagues convinced him that he would find more surgical opportunity in the city than down in the Minnesota farmland.

Thus in April 1873 he moved to St. Paul and established himself in partnership with another doctor there, leaving his family back in Rochester. This arrangement lasted a brief three months and no longer. Precisely what happened there no one seems to know for sure. There may have been more patients, but there were also a great many more doctors, including men who fancied themselves surgeons. Perhaps the little doctor had begun enjoying the local respect and deference of his Rochester patients more than he realized. Perhaps Mrs. Mayo grew weary of keeping a house and raising a family without her husband's presence and quietly exerted her influence. Whatever the reason, the doctor returned to Rochester quite abruptly one day, rented a new office above the Gossinger and Newtons' drugstore and resumed his practice in Rochester once and for all. At this time he was a man of fifty-four years. His son Will was a boy of twelve. Charlie was eight.

During the next few years Dr. Mayo's practice blossomed. He was rapidly gaining a reputation as a keen diagnostician, and doctors from the surrounding area began calling him in consultation on difficult medical problems. Finally, in 1880, he achieved a previously unrealized dream: He performed an abdominal operation on a woman to remove an ovarian tumor. Only eight such operations had ever been performed in Minnesota, all by other surgeons, and all but one ended in fatality. This operation was done in the patient's home under chloroform anesthesia. Dr. Mayo was assisted by his son-in-law, Dr. David Berkman, a veterinarian who had recently married his daughter Gertrude. Legend has it that young Will and Charlie were also in attendance, peeking through a crack in the door.

Certainly these were formative years for the boys. There seems never to have been any question that "the Mayo boys" would ultimately become doctors. Years later Dr. Will Mayo was quoted as saying: "We were raised into medicine the same as a farm boy is raised to farming." Yet most accounts one reads of their youth suggest that both boys slipped into medicine more by following their noses and their youthful curiosity than because of any special pressure from their imperious father. Perhaps Dr. Mayo simply assumed that of course his sons would be doctors—what else was there?—and never found it necessary to push. Or maybe even at that young age the boys were already sensing the exciting threshold of surgical progress upon which they were standing without ever having to be told.

Their preparation began early, and they had curiously mixed educations. As early as they could read, both boys were rooting out books from their father's library and taking anatomy lessons from the bones of the infamous Cut Nose that Dr. Mayo kept in a big iron kettle in his office. They became familiar with *Gray's Anatomy* and other anatomy books in the library. Will in particular was taken with a book of Paget's lectures on surgical pathology, in which he first encountered the name of John Hunter, one of the early students of gross pathology who was to become a hero to the boy. Oddly enough, neither of the brothers did particularly well in public school. Will disliked mathematics heartily and did only indifferently in other courses, while Charlie, coming later, hated the whole idea of school so much that he kept playing hooky and, once finally cured of that, devoted more time to mischief-making than study.

To balance this, the boys learned a great deal of botany and astronomy from their mother and physics and chemistry from their father. Both boys had their household chores to do, first in the big house in Rochester and then on the farm when the family had moved out there, but while Charlie enjoyed farming, Will hated every bit of it and soon got a job in a local Rochester drugstore to get away from it. Charlie continued to fiddle with mechanical things and, according to family legend, at the age of fourteen installed the first telephone in Rochester to connect his father's office with the farm home. Apparently their father was not overly impressed with the Rochester public school system either; each boy in his turn was withdrawn from high school after two years and placed in a private academy in the area designed to prepare youngsters for college.

Presently, of course, their direct contacts with medicine became more frequent. Both boys in turn were assigned the job of cleaning their father's office, taking care of his horses and driving him on his rounds. Ordinarily they would sit outside while the doctor saw his patient, but in cold weather he would allow them to come into the house so they could see the patient too. They learned how to roll bandages, apply plaster poultices, put on casts and similar jobs. When their father bought a new and expensive microscope, the boys learned how to fix bits of organ tissue into blocks with alcohol, cut and mount sections and study the slides at a time when the whole science of microscopic pathology was still in diapers. They watched their father doing autopsies at an early age; later they were allowed to assist at his operations in small ways, measuring and waxing the silk or linen sutures, threading them on needles and then sticking them through their coat lapels so their father could reach out for them whenever he needed one. Later still they were holding retractors and handling sponges.

Finally, in the fall of 1880, the time had come for the first fledgling to fly the nest: Will Mayo entered medical school. The place selected was the medical college at the University of Michigan, one of the few schools of the day with serious entrance requirements, a distinguished faculty of doctors who stressed clinical teaching in the medical sciences, a large chemistry laboratory available to medical students and the beginning of the first real University Hospital in the country.

The one-man Mayo medical practice in Rochester was about to become a two-man practice.

6

Rochester, Minnesota / *June 1979*

By 5:30 A.M. Tuesday morning Dr. Howard Norgaard was already up and dressed, looking out at the bright, cloudless Rochester sky. Already the air was shimmering with the promise of a scorching day ahead. Ungodly hot, these days, the surgeon reflected. Usually the real heat didn't hit until July and August.

He sipped coffee and nibbled toast without enthusiasm. For all his years of training and practice in cardiac surgery he still couldn't eat breakfast on the morning of a difficult case. Somehow the coiled-spring tension got to him every time; with anything more than coffee and toast he would be queasy and nauseated before he was an hour into his operation.

Still in his pajamas, he took the phone into his study and dialed a number. In thirty seconds his first assistant was on the line. "Well, Buzz? Where do we stand on the girl?"

"You haven't had a call all night, have you?"

"No, but I haven't slept much, either."

"She's looking good, sir. At least as good as we could expect. Charlie Hornby was in again just half an hour ago. She had a bad spell around two, a long run of ventricular premature beats, but then they settled down."

"So Charlie said we could go ahead?"

"He said we'd better go while we could and not try to fool around with too many pre-op studies, nice as they might be.

She's in as good shape as she's going to get, but he doesn't think she's going to hang around waiting too long."

"Then let's confirm the seven-o'clock time and get moving."

Norgaard hung up the receiver and dressed in the light cotton suit and open-necked shirt that he liked to wear these hot days, with a tie tucked into his side pocket. As he drove through the quiet, tree-shaded streets it seemed that most of the town was still asleep. Arriving at St. Mary's Hospital, he greeted a few early birds on the oncoming crew—a couple of OR nurses, a staff doctor and two Fellows coming over from the Clinic on the first shuttle bus. He took the elevator up to the operating-room floor, checked the call board of procedures listed for the day and walked into the doctors' dressing room.

His case was scheduled for Room 15, a room which, for some odd reason, he particularly liked for his open-heart procedures. It was not the most modern operating room in the hospital, nor the most spacious. In fact, it was downright cramped when his entire crew was crowded in there, together with monitoring equipment, heart-lung machine, anesthesia equipment and all. But for him there was a comfortable, almost old-fashioned feeling about the place, with its white tile on the walls up to shoulder height, cool green paint above that, white tile on the floor and swinging doors leading to the scrub rooms and corridor. Around two sides of the room, rising six feet above the operating theater, was an observers' gallery, with two tiers of benches accessible by way of a corridor on the floor above, open to the operating room and guarded by a barrier of three-inch brushed stainless-steel tubing. It was, Norgaard reflected, just the kind of operating room Will Mayo would have felt comfortable in. Hell, maybe Will Mayo *used* this operating room in the years before his death, for all he knew. Howard Norgaard had never bothered to find out.

The doctors' dressing room connected with the "clean areas" of the operating suite, forbidden to all but operating-room personnel. At his locker Dr. Norgaard slipped out of his street clothes and into a pajamalike blue-green scrub suit.

He put on a special pair of shoes which had never left the doctors' dressing room or operating room since the day he bought them. He had selected these "work shoes" very carefully to be easy on his feet while standing through surgical procedures that very often went ten and twelve hours without a break. (One during his training had gone on for twenty-two hours straight, he recalled, with the responsible surgeon taking only two ten-minute breaks to go to the john and wolf down a sandwich before rescrubbing and gowning to carry on.) He donned cloth booties over the operating shoes and then tugged on a blue-green cap, a procedure that always seemed to make his ears thrust out sideways and exaggerate the sharp, craggy features of his face.

Finally he tied a mask around his neck and stepped out into the doctors' lounge for a cup of coffee. He found his favorite lumpy, naugahyde chair over in one corner, stretched his legs out, put his head back, closed his eyes and made a conscious attempt to relax the tension developing in the muscles of his shoulders and neck.

He didn't go see the girl. He wouldn't ordinarily see his first surgical patient of the day anyway except in the operating room; his Fellows would have seen the patient earlier and called him if anything had happened during the night to alter his surgical plans. In fact, the first patient would ordinarily be in the anesthesia room or operating room already, undergoing final preparations for the surgery. But most especially, he hadn't wanted to see Manuela La Barca this morning, with her huge brown eyes that had watched him so distrustfully the night before and her frail, washed-out body like a porcelain doll in the bed. *A short lifetime of endless illness; three previous massive surgical insults, and now a fourth one coming up, with that narrow thread of life raveling far too thin by now*—the surgeon shook his head. He didn't have a good feeling about Manuela. *If only I could have been there the last time this was done*—

He saw Buzz Turnbull, his senior surgical Fellow, making his way across the room. The younger man poured coffee and sat down beside him. "Are they almost ready?" Norgaard asked.

"Pretty close," the younger man said, "Jerry'll page us when it's time to scrub."

"Was she still as scared as she was last night?"

"Hard to tell. She was pretty sleepy. But maybe Ed Ruiz got through to her. Just hearing someone speak her own language may have helped."

Norgaard nodded. "When we're finished, let's find a Spanish-speaking nurse to spend some time with her, even if she doesn't do anything else. Or maybe we can get one of the interpreters from over at the Clinic to help us keep tabs on what's bothering her. She can speak English, all right, but apparently she doesn't like to."

They sat sipping their coffee in silence for a long while. Then a quiet voice came from the wall speaker. "Dr. Norgaard, Room Fifteen please."

Norgaard glanced at his assistant. "I guess that's us," he said.

"Sounds like it."

"So let's get moving."

Only in retrospect did Howard Norgaard realize what an exceedingly long, exacting and tedious procedure it was, as technically difficult and physically draining as any operation he could remember. The operating room seemed already crammed with people and equipment when he and Turnbull arrived: the two scrub nurses, the circulating nurse and the back-up circulating nurse; Norgaard's second assistant surgeon as well as a third young man, a first-year surgical Fellow, supposedly on hand for back-up but mostly just to observe. In addition there was the anesthesiologist and his assistant, plus two technicians to help man the monitoring equipment and the heart-lung machine. In a great many medical centers the cardiac surgery was always performed by rigidly constituted teams who invariably operated together. At Mayo this was not always possible; the surgeons themselves would work as fixed teams in most cases, but the supporting personnel might vary more from case to case. But since all involved were so thoroughly and intensively trained, such mixing didn't matter too much.

In addition to the people on the operating floor, there

were four doctors up in the gallery this morning, gowned, capped and masked to observe the case. One was a young surgeon from Pierre, South Dakota, who often stopped in Rochester to observe surgery on his way home from trips to the East. He had heard from another surgeon that Dr. Norgaard might be doing a tough one this morning, and came in early to observe. Two other visitors were from Mobile, Alabama, vacationing in Minnesota and stopping by Mayo Clinic for the first time. The fourth man, Dr. Jorge Hernandez Aguilar, was the aging family physician who had been helping with Manuela's care for years and had come along with her and her parents on the plane from Mexico City the day before.

The gallery didn't exactly bother Dr. Norgaard, but he was not one for showmanship either. Unlike some of his surgical colleagues—the "prima donnas," as he regarded them a little scornfully—he refused to lecture and demonstrate to the gallery in the course of procedure, even though he knew it was a long-standing Mayo tradition to do so. Visiting surgeons had been coming here to observe surgery for three-quarters of a century. At first, of course, they had come to see Will and Charlie doing their pioneering operations, but as the Clinic and staff grew, other surgeons too were happy enough to step into the limelight. Not Howard Norgaard. He had learned long since that he was a single-minded surgeon. The work he did required his total absorption, without distractions, and he had built up something of a local reputation for being crusty and irritable in dealing with observers.

Now, aside from checking that everything was working as it should, Norgaard ignored the people and machinery in the room and concentrated his full attention on a small square of the patient's chest exposed among the sterile drapes. From the beginning it was a meticulous, painstaking, time-consuming job, dissecting through scar tissue from previous operations, with Buzz Turnbull across the table from him and the first-year Fellow close at his side—searching for landmarks that should have been there but couldn't be found any more because of previous scarring, making decisions again and again about what portion of bone to excise, what cartilage, what muscle tissue, working doggedly, waiting for a bleeder to stop, working, muttering to himself, working some more. Almost three hours alone were spent just opening the chest to expose the malfunctioning heart—and then the work *really* began. From time to time one of the others would pass on some information—the reading from a monitor, the blood-pressure level, the starting of another unit of blood, a change in anesthesia level—and he would nod and go on, more uneasy by the moment. *God, it was taking time!* Too much time, far more than he dared to take, and instinct was warning him that time was fast running out.

Then a technician muttered something in his ear and he knew his instinct had been right. He glanced at the monitor screen in alarm. "Damn!" he said softly. "We'd better get her on the machine and fast."

Buzz Turnbull looked up. "Trouble?"

"She's going out on us, that's all. Let's get those cannulas ready and *move*. We can finish the dissection later." He looked over his shoulder. "Charlie Hornby's on the floor somewhere. Will somebody please get him in here? We're going to need him."

Without a wasted moment then, they turned to the desperate task, inserting the blood-conducting cannulas in the proper places and shifting the child's entire heart and lung function over to the heart-lung machine so that her fast-failing heart could be stopped. "Let's at least get pressures in the heart chambers," Norgaard said. "We've got to know what we're starting with. We know that aortic valve is shot, and Christ only knows what else, but we need baseline pressures or we won't know what we've accomplished."

It took time, but they did it, and after long tense minutes Norgaard got the nod that the heart-lung machine was functioning. Manuela's blood was now being oxygenated and circulated throughout her body without requiring the pumping aid of her heart, so that now, at least, its feeble, irregular beat could be temporarily stopped.

From then on Norgaard and Buzz Turnbull worked together like a well-rehearsed team, first completing the dissection of scar tissue that remained to be done, then proceeding to open the heart itself. With a "dry heart" to work on, they could identify the damaged valve structures, study them to see what had gone wrong and what had to be done to remove and replace them. Dr. Charles Hornby had come in and stood by throughout, rigged up in cap, mask and gown and looking as ridiculously awkward as only a pediatrician can look in an operating room. He peered over Norgaard's shoulder, grunted approval of the way the heart-lung machine was operating and the patient was looking. "She's nice and pink right now, Howie," he said.

"Yeah. So far we're okay, if she didn't throw a clot to the brain back there when she nearly went out."

"The EEG looks okay."

"Good. But would you mind sticking around till we pull her off the machine and start her heart up again? I don't know *what's* going to happen then."

"Don't worry, I'll be here," Hornby said.

Six and a half hours after they had started the procedure the repair and valve replacement was completed, the heart-lung machine support was discontinued and the child's heartbeat restarted. At first it faltered and then, miraculously, both heart and lungs began working for themselves again in a regular steady rhythm. Hornby ordered some intravenous medication given, hovering over the monitors like a small rumpled vulture. Norgaard checked the new pressure figures for the heart chambers and began looking happier than he had all day. "You know, Buzz," he said quietly, "we might just possibly sneak by on this one, with a little bit more luck. Let's get going on this closure now."

Two hours and a quarter later, it was finally, incredibly over, and the surgeons walked out into the corridor as preparations were made to shift the still-sleeping girl into the intensive-care recovery room. Charlie Hornby followed her along; he would stay nearby until she could be moved back upstairs to the cardiac intensive-care unit. Norgaard buzzed for a stenographer and stood in the middle of the corridor to dictate his extensive operative note, a detailed and technical description of everything that had been done in the operating room. By the time he finished dressing it would be typed up and ready for his signature. Meanwhile he found Buzz Turnbull in the doctors' lounge gulping down a sandwich and four cartons of milk. "Okay, Buzz, it's all yours," Norgaard said. "I'll be back in time for that case at three-thirty. Meanwhile, I'd better go talk to this girl's parents."

Buzz looked up with an odd expression. "Are you going to tell them she's cured?"

"No way," Norgaard said. "I'm going to tell them she's still alive and be damned glad I can tell them that. I'm also going to tell them to pray, because that girl is going to need it. She's got one bloody rough road ahead of her in the next few days."

"Just as an example," I said, "what would be the total cost to a patient for an open-heart operation here? And how would the patient pay for it?"

I was talking to Mr. John J. See, the senior comptroller for the Mayo Clinic, sitting in his small, stuffy office on the second floor of the Mayo Building on a hot June afternoon. At that time I had not even heard of the case of Manuela La Barca; and indeed, as a matter of fixed policy, there was no time that Mr. See or anyone else associated with Mayo Clinic would discuss *any* individual patient with an outsider, not even off the record, except in the vaguest generalities. "A patient came here once" or "I remember a woman" was as far as they would go.

Mr. See spread his hands at my question. "Open-heart surgery? It all depends on the nature of the case, the amount of pre- and post-operative care required, the specific services that have to be rendered and so forth," he said. "Even then I couldn't tell you with absolute certainty because there would be the hospital bills that would never show up on our billings."

"But I thought the hospitals were a part of the institution," I said.

"Heavens, no. At least, not in any financial sense. St. Mary's Hospital and Rochester Methodist are each separately owned, separately administered and separately financed. They set their own charges and send their own hospital bills. True, Clinic doctors make up the entire medical staffs of both hospitals, exclusively. We provide them with resident physicians and use them as teaching hospitals. We provide them with Emergency Room doctors, and the Clinic also does all the laboratory and X-ray work for both hospitals. This greatly simplifies the hospitals' cost accounting, since they can concentrate on housekeeping and nursing-care functions alone, without having to worry about all the other things most hospitals have to provide. It also means a considerable economy to the patient, too. It wouldn't make sense, for example, to have three huge clinical laboratory and X-ray facilities located within the same city mile. That wouldn't provide any better service, but it could easily lead to skyrocketing costs."

Mr. See sat back in his swivel chair. He was a small gray-haired, slightly balding man who looked as if he might have been tucked away in some corner of the place for the last forty-five years. I had met him a few minutes earlier in the cool, spacious lobby of the Mayo Building, and he had conducted me up to his low-ceilinged office by way of a staff elevator. "To get back to your original question, a coronary artery bypass procedure, for example, in a patient who was not so terribly sick that he needed weeks of stabilization before the operation might end up costing, say, twelve to fourteen thousand dollars in all for hospital and Clinic combined. *Our* billing would show his Clinic workup, any consultations he had, his laboratory work, his angiocardiography, surgeons' and assistants' fees for the procedure, the anesthesiologists' fees—anything connected with the Clinic. The hospital would bill separately for his hospital room and board, the use of the operating room and specialized equipment, the use of the recovery room, intensive care as needed and any other purely hospital-related items. Then the patient would make arrangements with us for payment of the Clinic's bill."

"That's a pretty staggering sum of money," I said. "So how would he pay it?"

"Any way that works out best," Mr. See said.

"You mean for the Clinic?"

He gave me a reproachful look. "I mean for the patient, first; then for the Clinic. Obviously, cash on the barrelhead would be best for the Clinic—but we would hardly expect that."

"Well, I suppose you'd bill his Blue Cross or whatever and any major medical he carried," I said.

"We would provide his insurance company—or companies—with all the information they would need to process his claim," Mr. See said. "We would even help him with follow-up, if necessary, to collect from the insurance company whatever it would pay. The patient could assign payment to us, or receive it himself at his option. However—" Mr. See raised a finger—"the Mayo Clinic has no contract with Blue Cross or Blue Shield or Medicare or any other medical insurance organization. We never have had. What we *do* have is an unspoken contract with the patient to provide him with medical services for a certain fee, and it is *his* obligation to *us* to pay that fee, whatever the insurance company may allow against it."

The man spread his hands. "Sometimes that leads to problems—maybe unavoidable problems. Sometimes when a patient's treatment is completed he gives his insurance company number to the business office and figures, 'Here you are; they're supposed to pay the bill. I wash my hands of it.' So we attach our bill to the claim form and answer follow-up queries and so forth and then some day, presently, the insurance carrier sends a check—for sixty percent of the bill. So then we write the patient and remind him that he still owes forty percent, and the patient is very upset. 'Why are you billing *me?*' he wants to know. 'My insurance is supposed to pay.' The truth is, that patient has never once even *looked* at his medical insurance policy, much less read it through, so he doesn't *know* that the insurance pays only a percentage of charges.

"Well, he may be annoyed at the insurance company, but he's liable to be hopping mad at us, and sometimes there's lots of bad feeling before we finally collect. I think maybe this is how so many stories originate about how heartless and greedy and depersonalized doctors and clinics and hospitals are, how unfair they are, how high their fees are—because nobody ever *told* the patient that his insurance doesn't cover the full amount of charges. Well, we combat the problem the best we can by sending the full bill to the patient as well as the insurance company. The patient has right there on paper what his bill to us is and he knows it's *his* bill to *us*. If Blue Cross pays sixty percent of it one way or another, he feels he's sixty percent ahead, not forty percent behind." Mr. See shook his head. "It's been that way here ever since Will and Charlie decided they had to set up some kind of organized billing system instead of the weird, haphazard fee system the old man used to use."

"If this is true," I said, "you surely must make some sort of extended payment arrangements for patients who don't have the whole fee on hand at once."

"Certainly we do. In fact, we'll cooperate in just about any way we can think of to enable a patient to pay his bill, however big it may be, with as little distress as possible—and we don't assess finance charges, either. Of course there's one advantage to fame: A lot of people who come here don't have to worry about how they're going to pay their medical bills because they've got more money than they know what to do with. But a great many more are just plain, ordinary lower-middle-class people with small medical insurance policies and not much reserve. Others are just about penniless, and we have to make adjustments in our bills. But not very often."

"Don't you have an awful lot of defaults?" I said.

"Not really." Mr. See put his fingers together and stared at the ceiling. "With a quarter of a million patients through here last year, our overall collection ratio was right around ninety-six percent. That's not *too* bad."

"You mean you collect *ninety-six percent* of all your billings?"

"That's right."

"Well, you must be doing *something* right," I said. "What kind of financial screening do you put all those people through before you let them into the place?"

"We don't screen them at all," See said.

"No little discussion with some nice young lady at a desk

downstairs? No questions about employment or income or bank accounts or savings or anything like that?"

See laughed and shook his head. "Not a single question," he said. "The patient doesn't even go *near* the business office until his treatment is concluded."

My face must have given me away, because See laughed again. "I really mean it," he said. "I know it sounds a little bizarre—or at least awfully reckless—but you've got to understand the background of this place. There was a time, years ago, back in nineteen-seventeen or so, when Dr. Will and Dr. Charlie wanted to establish a formal relationship between the Mayo Foundation for Medical Education and Research and the University of Minnesota Medical School. To finance it, the Mayos offered the University a free gift of one and a half million dollars, which was quite a heap of money in those days. You might have thought the state would jump at the chance, but Will and Charlie had enemies, especially among the medical people up in the Cities, and all of a sudden there were all kinds of nasty rumors going around about how this pair of greedy surgeons down in Rochester were trying some kind of takeover of the Medical School, about how they figured to carry a lot of state money down to Rochester for their own benefit and a lot of patients as well, and so on into the night."

See stretched his legs out alongside his desk. "Well, Dr. Charlie was too good-natured to get sore, but Will had all of these rumors he could take, and when the time arrived for debate and vote on the matter in the State Senate Committee on Education, he was hopping mad. So the evening of the committee meeting he went up to the Cities to speak, just throwing off sparks, and he told those boys how it was at the Mayo Clinic. He told them that he and his brother had built a great medical institution out of nothing by virtue of hard work and good medicine and certain high ideals they'd learned from their father. He told them that he and Charlie had never yet turned anybody away from their doors who needed treatment, regardless of cost, and they never asked a patient if he had the price, and they weren't about to start asking, either. And as for him and Charlie being greedy, he told them: 'If we wanted money, we have it. We have never taken notes at the Clinic. No mortgage has ever been given on a home to pay a bill there. We never sue. Thirty percent of our patients are charity cases. About twenty-five percent pay barely the cost of treatment.' "

Mr. See stood up. "That was back in nineteen-seventeen, mind you. Of course we're very much bigger now. We treat a whole lot more patients, and things are a lot more expensive, and fees are a lot higher than they were in those days. Inevitably some things, mostly minor things, have changed—but not very much, when you get down to it. And not the basic principles those two men established seventy-five years or more ago."

He picked up a three-inch-thick stack of computer read-out sheets. "If you want a couple of months of fascinating reading, you might go through this—it's our fee schedule. Every service and procedure available at the Clinic from a simple urinalysis to a carotid artery thromboendarterectomy is listed in there with identifying numbers. Every day each patient's charges are posted in the computer and ultimately come down here for final accuracy check before a print-out is made. Come take a look."

He threw open a door and we walked out into a room the size of Yankee Stadium (it seemed) filled with row upon row of computer keyboards, each operated by an extremely busy young woman or man and each equipped with a television read-out screen. Each girl had in her hand what looked like a long narrow flashlight or stylus connected to a wire and was going down a read-out of charges on the television screen, comparing it to a stack of papers beside her; each time she touched an item on the television screen with the stylus, the item vanished. "It's intensive work," Mr. See told me, "and they've got to be accurate, comparing each charge against the patient's record. It wears these people out; they work only two hours at a time and then take a long rest break—but we end up with virtually no error and the patient gets a detailed, itemized chronological record of everything that was done while he was here. If he has to bill an insurance company, we provide him with an additional copy of his read-out to staple to the insurance form. The names of the doctors he's seen, the diagnoses all properly coded, everything the insurance company could reasonably need to verify a claim without wasting time on the long, three-page, type-written reports some insurance outfits would like to make you fill out for them."

He excused himself then, pleading a luncheon committee meeting, conducting me to the staff elevator and pushing the right button to get me to the lobby. As I joined the crowd down below, I walked around to Station E, the wing of the lobby where patients are sent when their treatment is completed to pick up their bills and make arrangements for payment. As at each of the other lobby stations, there were several hundred padded straight chairs in the section facing a long counter with some twenty partitioned areas like tellers' cages.

I sat down to watch. As each patient arrived, the receptionist directed him to a numbered window according to who was least busy. The clerk at the counter took the patient's name and asked him to have a seat—but they weren't kept sitting long. Within ten minutes at the longest they were called back to the counter to receive their bills. Some wrote checks on the spot. Some held lengthy conversations with their "tellers." Still others went farther down the room where half a dozen young women at desks were consulting with patients about insurance forms and claims. In most cases the patients were in and out of Section E within a maximum of twenty minutes. None that I saw appeared gray of face, tearful or shocky as they walked away, and none of them shrieked and fainted upon presentation of their bills. Most, in fact, looked remarkably cheerful, more interested in telling Aunt Mabel about their new heart pills than in complaining about their charges.

Finally I went on my way. I was only beginning to comprehend how the Mayo Clinic could be seeing an average of 1,000 new patients each day of the week except Saturdays and Sundays from one end of the year to the other with anything approaching efficiency. One answer, obviously, was that wherever purely mechanical functions were involved—

routine business-office functions, for example—the skids were greased in every possible way.

Roger Barton encountered the diagnostic end of things at the Mayo Clinic with a vengeance on Tuesday, his second day in Rochester, and he wasn't sure whether to be angry or pleased. On the one hand, he was raked over more thoroughly than ever before in his life—but he had also never before felt quite so much like a very small cog in an enormous machine, and he couldn't help but wonder if he might be chewed to mincemeat if he happened to fall out of step at one point or another along the way.

When he'd left Dr. DeVore the previous afternoon the receptionist at the E-14 desk had handed him back his brown paper wallet. "Now don't lose this," she said. "It's got all your appointments in it for tomorrow. You look them over tonight and be down at Desk C in the Conrad Hilton Building tomorrow morning at seven o'clock."

He had heard about the infamous Desk C from other patients he had talked to, where demoniac blood-guzzlers rammed tenpenny nails into your arms and committed all manner of other indignities upon your person—and then charged you for it. That evening in his room he had inspected the contents of his brown paper wallet with extra care, as well as the other goodie the woman had handed him: a small brown paper bag containing a urine specimen bottle, with directions for collecting the specimen and depositing it in one of the collection baskets stationed around the lobby even before seven o'clock next day. He saw that his appointment at the Conrad Hilton Building was indeed for the collection of blood samples and discovered to his horror that he was to have nothing to eat or drink after ten o'clock that evening until those blood samples had been drawn. The instructions even went to the extreme of telling him that if he brushed his teeth in the morning he must rinse his mouth without swallowing and that a morning cup of coffee was definitely a no-no.

Well, Roger thought, that was ridiculous. How could a person function without coffee and breakfast in the morning?

And at 7:00 A.M., for God's sake! They were just putting on a show that they were doing something special with all these fancy instructions. Just throwing their weight around. But on the other hand—he paused and scratched his chin. Maybe the crafty bastards were trying to trap him. Maybe they could look at those blood samples they were going to take and somehow *tell* if he'd eaten something before the sample was taken and get the word back to Dr. DeVore. Roger grumbled and groused and muttered to himself and felt put upon, but in the end he did *not*, in fact, have anything to eat or drink after 10:00 P.M.; he *did*, in fact, rinse out his mouth next morning without swallowing; and he *did*, in fact, present himself at Desk C in the Conrad Hilton Building at 7:00 A.M. with his stomach rumbling like Mt. Etna but quite empty of either coffee or toast.

He nearly didn't make it after all. He had carefully allowed time to choose the proper summer ensemble with which to adorn himself in order to make a suitable impression on the young ladies he felt sure he was going to encounter that day. *After all, you can't go around looking like a farmer,* he thought, *and then, with all these females around, there's no telling what you might end up doing before the day is out.* But with that finally done and himself properly launched from his hotel room, he had promptly gotten lost in the Clinic subway system trying to find Desk C.

He'd chosen that route because he'd heard the subways were air-conditioned and the day looked like a scorcher outside. He had started briskly down the underground walkway from the Kahler, reached the central arcade under the Mayo Building lobby, took a turn and suddenly found himself in the basement of Rochester Methodist Hospital. Retracing his steps, he took another turn and ended up in the Plummer Building. Ignoring the numerous "You Are Here" signs posted frequently on the walls to help addled old ladies (or even bright young men like Roger Barton) find out where they were and where they were going, Roger plunged on, down one corridor after another, getting nowhere. He was beginning to feel ridiculous, starting up what seemed to be the same corridor for the third time, when a matronly woman in a nurse's uniform stopped and asked if she could help him.

"I'm supposed to go to Desk C," Roger said, feeling foolish.

"Oh yes. Well, you go back to the big arcade where you passed the drugstore, you remember, and then take the first corridor to the left and that will take you straight to Desk C. And oh yes—" she pointed to the paper bag he was clutching—"*that* goes into that cart over there against the wall. The girls make a pickup every ten minutes."

He finally found himself in a bright carpeted corridor with potted plants stationed at regular intervals. Many people seemed to be going the same direction that he was, including gentlemen on crutches and ladies in wheelchairs. Soon he emerged from the corridor into an enormous skylighted room with a large reception desk to his left, bearing a sign that said: DESK C. He rushed up to the receptionist like a man who's just found water on the desert. "Here I am," he said.

"That's *very* good, sir," the woman said. "May I have your appointment wallet, please?"

"My what?"

"That little brown paper wallet. It tells us what to do now that you are here."

He slapped his pockets in a moment of rising panic, then found the wallet in one of his side jacket pockets. He handed it to the girl, who took a slip from it, stamped it with a time stamp and tucked it into a slot in her desk. "Fine," she said. "I'll give your wallet back when you're through here. Now if you'll just take a seat and wait until your name is called, please."

Seats were in good supply in this huge room—there must have been 500—and two-thirds of them were already full. They all faced a large semicircular wall punctuated by a whole series of doors, each painted a different color. One door was blue, one was green, one orange, one yellow, one violet. From time to time a very young girl in a white aide's uniform would emerge from one or another of these colored doors, pick up a hand microphone from a rack by the door and call out seven or eight names. When the names were Anderson or Peterson or Henderson, the girls had no problem. They didn't even do so badly with names such as Heinrichner or Karshmann or Holtzenberger. It was when they ran into names like Boyarskevitch or Hashokito or al Fatimah or Poisson that they faltered. In fact, the latter-named person, a dignified elderly gentleman, marched up to his summoner and said, very loudly, "Young woman, I wish you to know that my name is *not* pronounced 'poison,' as in 'arsenic.'"

As these clusters of seven or eight patients were recruited, they were promptly escorted behind the colored doors. Roger noticed with a certain growing alarm that none of them ever seemed to come out again. To divert his mind he looked around the huge room in which he was sitting. Obviously the architect who had designed the Conrad Hilton Building and its subway connection with the Clinic building had exercised some imagination: This "underground" room on the subway level had no building above it at all. Much of the ceiling was an enormous skylight surrounded by a well-kept garden. Compared to the sterile interior waiting rooms in the Clinic building and the gloomy corridors of the old Plummer Building, this was a refreshing change for the people sitting here, especially considering the unspeakable torments many imagined they were going to suffer before they got out. Roger, of course, knew that they were only going to take blood samples, yet his own uneasiness became so intense as he waited that he missed his own name when it was called and it had to be repeated twice.

He was summoned by an attractive young lady from behind the green door, which set his imagination working fiercely. Inside, however, was merely an anteroom with benches where he and others were asked to sit down. One by one the others in the group disappeared into a room to the rear, never again to emerge. Finally he too was called, to be greeted in the back room by a gray-haired matron who seemed to know exactly what she was doing and a very young girl who looked as though she didn't. After a bit of banter about where he came from and how he liked Rochester (how *could* one like Rochester, for God's sake?) and whether he'd had any breakfast that morning, which he answered rather belligerently in the negative, his arm was out, his sleeve was up, the tourniquet was on and the matronly lady was pointing to his elbow region and saying to the young girl, "Right *there*."

Roger preferred not to watch, but it was all over, it seemed, almost before it had begun. He was appalled at the whole row of test tubes filled with blood taken from his arm, but he followed the matron's directions to slip his jacket back on, go out through a door to the rear of the small cubicle and follow a corridor back to the receptionist at Desk C to pick up his appointment wallet and receive instructions for his next waystop. Sure enough, the wallet was waiting for him at the desk.

His next appointment was for an electrocardiogram to be taken on the first floor of the Plummer Building. This journey he chose to make overland, going up to the main lobby of the Mayo Building and out the big glass east door, dodging an attendant helping a little old lady in a wheelchair through the door and stepping briskly to avoid the steady stream of taxicabs and hotel vans driving up to the curb under the overhang to discharge patients. Across the street he went into the central lobby of the Plummer Building, a beautiful old building of the vintage of the 1920s, with its handsome marble paneling and a four-winds compass in colored terrazzo tile set in the middle of the lobby floor. The first-floor corridors were pleasantly dark and cool in the growing heat of the day, with ancient wood-and-leather chairs along either side. All in all, there was a pleasant air of musty age and gentility about the place reminiscent of earlier times when, perhaps, the Mayo Clinic was less shiny, less crowded and less hurried.

All this was lost on Roger Barton, who was realizing with a sense of betrayal that this EKG appointment was following so hard on the heels of the previous one that there was no opportunity to stop for a bite of breakfast in between—nor any place to stop, either, for that matter.

At the EKG lab he was kept waiting only briefly. Then a pleasant young woman took him back to one of several cubicles with a screened corner serving as a dressing room. He was told to disrobe to his underwear, put on a paper gown and sit on the large padded table until she returned. Roger did so, reflecting upon what a very attractive young woman she was and what a damned dull evening it was going to be unless he got busy and started tilling the fields. Her attractiveness seemed tempered with a certain reserve, however, when she returned ten minutes later, placed him out flat on his back on the table and began attaching the EKG wires. In fact, she seemed quite distant and unresponsive to a couple of preliminary humorous sallies, interrupting him in mid-sentence to ask him to please stop talking while she was running the machine, and then before he knew it she was busy wrapping up the leads again, the EKG taken.

"I say, let me have a look at that," Roger said, pointing to the long strip of tape with squiggles on it.

"Oh, your doctor will tell you all about it," the girl said.

"Well, look—how about—uh—like maybe dinner somewhere this evening?" Roger was feeling ridiculous in his paper gown and undershorts.

"Oh, I'm afraid I couldn't." The girl was pleasantly regretful, but she already had an engagement. In fact, she seemed to have a *very* active social life, booked full every evening of the week—and the next—and the next. "Now when you get dressed," she said, "just go out to the reception desk and pick up your appointment wallet—" and off she went with the cardiogram in her hand.

At the reception desk he asked the woman, "Where do I go next?"

"Over to the third floor of the Mayo Building for your chest X ray. They're expecting you right now."

Roger cleared his throat. "You know, I haven't had any breakfast yet," he said.

The woman laughed heartily. "Yes, isn't it awful? Some people just shrivel away into nothing before they get through here."

Since there was obviously going to be no sympathy from *this* quarter, Roger went across to the Mayo Building, had a chest X ray taken, both a front view and a side view (to which he objected, "I've never heard of taking a chest X ray from the side before") and then peppered the technician (a man) with questions about how much extra radiation exposure he had received from two views of chest, and would he get to see the films, and how much shielding there was in the walls of the X-ray department and so forth and so on until he suddenly realized that the technician wasn't even listening, and he decided to give up.

By the time the X rays were finished it was getting well along in the morning and Roger very nearly decided to pass up the next appointment—something called Pulmonary Function Lab—in favor of a nice solid breakfast of sausage, eggs and hash browns with a short stack of pancakes on the side. But he remembered what Dr. DeVore had said about the importance of the respiratory study, especially considering his heavy and long-standing cigarette smoking, so he turned up at the designated place on the third floor of the Plummer Building only twelve minutes late.

A young woman immediately escorted him into a small room virtually packed with machines, breathing tubes the size of vacuum-cleaner hoses, oxygen tanks and a large computer with a visual screen, a keyboard and a number of ink styluses that made a succession of colored lines on a broad sheet of graph paper that rolled out of the machine.

"Well," the woman said, "I see that you're late, so we're going to have to get right busy. We've got lots of work to do in the next hour."

"But I haven't had any breakfast," Roger said. "I'm liable to fall over on my face if I have to do any work."

"Oh, that's all right," the woman said cheerfully. "We'll just pick you back up again if you do."

She seemed to be smiling at him, but something in her voice hauled Roger up like a reined-in horse. This was a different breed of cat than he had encountered elsewhere around this place. Like every other female he'd seen here, she was more than just presentably attractive: red-blond hair done in a bun in the back, just a trace of eye makeup, a touch of perfume—but this woman was older, perhaps in her early thirties, and the smile did not reach up to her eyes—a pair of very cold, very disinterested ice-blue eyes. This woman was 100 percent business, here to get a job done—in Roger's case, it seemed, a rather unpleasant job—and there was going to be no nonsense about it. If a smiling façade would help her get the job done better and faster, then fine, she would wear a smiling façade, but she was going to get the job done whether Roger liked it or not. In fact, something suggested that she couldn't care less whether Roger liked it or not.

The process was *not* particularly pleasant and required almost continuous hard work on Roger's part. She scooted him from one breathing machine to another, first just measuring his lung capacity, how much he could breathe in and how much he could blow out in so much time, then going on to accelerated breathing exercises. Here she sat in front of him on a stool, telling him when to breathe, first slowly, then steadily faster and faster and faster, watching him with that tight little smile of hers, counting out the breaths the way a coxswain calls the strokes in a racing shell. When he couldn't breathe any deeper or faster, she urged him on mercilessly: "Come on now! You can do better than that! Deeper! More breaths! Blow it out harder! Faster now! Faster!" While he rested briefly between sessions, she pecked away at the computer keyboard, checked the tracings, deliberately placing herself so that he couldn't see them, then moving him on to another machine.

Presently they came to the step-test apparatus. She placed yet another breathing-machine mouthpiece in his mouth and a padded clip on his nose and had him start stepping up two steps and back down two steps, beating the pace on the support rail with her hand, making him move faster and faster until his tongue was hanging out. At one point he didn't think he could go on, but she gave him that tight, contemptuous little smile and said, "Just five more minutes," so that he had the joy of watching the second hand on the big wall clock creep around while she continued to harangue him.

Only once during the whole hour did he venture a question. After the first step-test she let him rest—so long by the clock—checking his pulse and his recovery from huffing and puffing. Then she got a little mechanical aerosol vaporizer and asked if he had ever had any allergic problem with Isuprel, a bronchial dilator. He hadn't, and he had certainly used it enough, so she gave him a standardized dose. She waited a few moments for it to take effect, then said, "Now let's do the step-test again and see if that doesn't improve your performance a little," as if his performance without it had been lousy.

He did the test again and then, when she went to the computer to look at the graph, he said, "Well, did it help any?"

She looked at him with those cold eyes. "What was your impression?" she asked.

"Well, I thought it helped some, but I couldn't be sure," Roger said.

"Then I guess the proof is in the pudding, isn't it?" she said and gave him that tight little smile again. "Now if you'll just step over here . . ." She led him through the last few procedures, ripped off the graph paper and rolled it into a tube and then said, "Okay, that's it. Your doctor will get all the reports." And just like that, he found himself standing out in the hall.

Only later did it strike him just what it was that woman had reminded him of: certain expensive prostitutes of his experience, with gorgeous, perfect bodies but icy cold, icily efficient, there to get the job done whether the "patient" happened to like the process or not, and when your time was up, bud, piss off. Except, of course, they had never sent reports to his doctor.

By this time it was almost noon, and Roger's next appointment, the blood-pressure lab, was not until 2:00, so he found his way back to the Elizabethan Room at the Kahler and made up for his lost breakfast with three double bourbons, herring in wine sauce, a modest twelve-ounce porterhouse steak, blood rare and well salted, and a half bottle of a rather nice Beaujolais, lighthearted in spirit but amusing in its assertiveness. As he lurched across the street at 2:00 to find the blood-pressure lab in the Mayo Building, he reflected that if they wanted him relaxed for his blood-pressure test, they were going to have him relaxed.

Or so he thought. Walking into the blood-pressure lab was like stepping into another world. A tiny blond girl escorted him into a small, quiet room with no windows, dimly lit by indirect lighting around the edges of the ceiling. In the room was a comfortable padded armchair and footrest; beside one chair arm stood a machine. Soft, soothing music was playing. The girl took his jacket, then rolled up his sleeve and took his blood pressure with an ordinary cuff, just as it had been taken in doctors' offices a thousand times before. Then she wrapped another cuff around his arm. "Now the machine will do it," she said. "You relax but try not to doze off. Every five minutes for the next half hour the cuff will inflate automatically and the machine will record your blood pressure. I'll be in later to rescue you."

Roger leaned back in the chair, but he did not relax. He found that his eyes were resting directly on a large wall clock with a sweep second hand—some enterprising clock salesman must have sold the Mayo Clinic 10,000 of those wall clocks—and as he watched the clock he waited for the first pressure reading. It was like watching grass grow. The second hand inched around the clock face once, then twice. Roger peered at his own watch, certain that the wall clock had to be running slow. Then he began to get nervous about what the cuff would feel like when it inflated. *Tight? Too tight?* Suddenly the cuff began inflating a full forty-five seconds before he thought it was due, and Roger jumped a foot out of the chair. As it started deflating again he heard the machine making a rhythmic click-click-click sound, very audible and very loud. He craned his head around, trying to see what it was doing. At one point it seemed that the machine skipped a click, and he looked again, getting panicky. Was that his *heartbeat* he was hearing?

Suddenly and inexplicably he began wheezing as if an asthma attack were starting. *So then what do I do? How am I going to get that girl in here so I can get my medicine out of my jacket? Just let out a bellow?* Now, if that little blonde would just come and sit on his lap while this was going on, he thought, maybe he could quiet down a bit—but somehow he had the feeling that the little blonde was *not* going to come sit on his lap.

He waited, keyed up as a cornered rabbit, for the second five-minute countdown, growing more and more apprehensive during the final seconds and again starting violently when the cuff began to inflate. Yes, by God, that sometimes-irregular click-click-click *was* his heartbeat! *So what does that missed beat mean? Are they going to find something wrong with my ticker, too? Why did I ever let myself come to this dump in the first place?*

As he waited for the third reading, he started another cheery train of thought. What if they found out that he *did* have high blood pressure? What would he have to do then? Lose a lot of weight? Go on some yucky string-bean diet? Cut out salt? Hell, he couldn't *live* without salt. Quit the smoking? Quit the drinking? God! Maybe quit the women too? Start taking that blood-pressure medicine that fixes you so you can't get it up any more? He'd heard about *that* stuff from a guy in Rotary and I mean, like, *he* couldn't make it any way at all. Roger leaped as the cuff inflated again.

It ended up being the longest thirty minutes Roger Barton had ever spent in his life. As soon as he was discharged he rushed over to his hotel room, took out his own blood-pressure cuff and measured his blood pressure. 120/80. But the valve was still sticking. *And I don't suppose you can buy another one anywhere in town,* he thought. *At least not without a doctor's prescription.*

His final appointment before seeing Dr. DeVore that afternoon was with a doctor in the Ear, Nose and Throat Department—an elderly and kindly man named MacMichael who peered at him over the tops of a pair of "foxy grandpa" half-glasses and seemed to smile an honest smile when he smiled, which was frequently. "Dr. DeVore wanted me to have a look at your nose and see if there's anything we can do about this obstruction that's bothering you. I'll need you to sit back in this examining chair now."

Roger had had these examinations before and they had always been murder. This one was different. The man was incredibly smooth. He knew *exactly* what he was doing and he knew how to do it with dispatch. Nothing he did took very long, and nothing that he did hurt—yet when he was through Roger sensed that he had never before had such a thorough examination of his nose and throat as the one Dr. Mac-Michael had just performed in a brief twenty minutes.

When the old gentleman had finished he sat back on a stool set low enough that he had to look up at Roger to talk. "Of course you do smoke a very great deal," he said, almost as if to himself, "and it shows."

"Shows?" Roger said.

"The erythema—that raw, red chronic irritation of the membranes in the throat and nose. We almost always see that in smokers. And you may well be having some degree of allergic reaction to one of the medicines you've been taking, as Dr. DeVore suggests. There are some things we can do to sort *that* out quickly enough." The doctor tilted his head and looked up at the patient. "The thing *I* wonder is how much real trouble you actually have with your nose."

"Well, it bothers me," Roger said, a little lamely.

"Constantly? Or just occasionally?"

"Well, a little bit every day, especially when I lie down to sleep on my back."

"Every day? Or just some days?"

"Maybe three or four days a week."

"To a minor degree," the doctor added.

"I guess you'd say that," Roger conceded.

"Well, you do have real physical nasal obstruction," MacMichael said. "It's commonly known as a deviated septum. The little strip of cartilage separating one side of the nose from the other gets pushed over to one side, almost blocking off one nostril, so all the air comes in the other. This leads to a certain amount of mouth breathing, which is irritating, and some drying of the open nostril, so that the body reacts by creating more mucus. Your septum is deviated, and it's undoubtedly contributing to your problem."

Aha, Roger thought, *the crafty old fox! Get you off guard and then slip you the news.* "And that sort of thing has to be corrected by surgery—is that what you're saying?"

"Well, it *can* be," Dr. MacMichael said. "But I don't think I'd recommend it in your case."

Roger looked up, blinking. "You wouldn't?"

"I don't think so."

"But why not? I thought you guys were big on surgery around here."

The doctor laughed. "Well, there's surgery and then there's surgery," he said. "If you had acute appendicitis within forty miles of this place, we'd whisk you into the operating room so fast you couldn't even squeak. But this is a little different."

The doctor smiled. "We like patients to be *happy* with our surgery, and we like it to do some good. And frankly, removing a deviated septum isn't the most satisfactory surgery in the world. It's a pretty unpleasant experience for the patient, hung up with this big uncomfortable nasal pack in place for days after the operation, and the risk of bleeding, and the risk of infection . . ." The doctor grimaced. "And then the results aren't always what one hopes for, either. Sometimes it works pretty well, but other times it just doesn't help that much. Of course, if a patient were having an enormous amount of trouble and nothing else seemed to help at all, we'd be obliged to consider surgery. But for you there are a number of more conservative things that might do the job as well or better. Personally, I think the allergy angle is the most promising." The doctor stood up and helped Roger down from the examining chair. "I'll be talking to Dr. DeVore immediately about my recommendations. I know he has some testing planned for you tomorrow, and I see from your appointment wallet that you're to be seeing him briefly at four this afternoon. For what it's worth, I think you're in good hands. He'll take good care of you."

Roger did see Dr. DeVore at four, but the interview was very brief. "Too early to have many reports back," the doctor said, "but we need to home in on this blood pressure of yours. It's way out of line."

Roger told the doctor about his trials in the blood-pressure lab but the doctor merely laughed. "You'll do better on a repeat run tomorrow," he said. "Even more important, we want you to start this very afternoon collecting a twenty-four-hour urine sample and a twenty-four-hour sputum sample. You pick up your appointment wallet at the front desk and they'll explain the whole schedule for tomorrow and then send you down to Desk C to get the containers for these specimens and the directions that go with them." He looked up sharply at Roger. "Follow the directions, my friend. They're very important. Then by tomorrow afternoon we should be able to do some reporting to you and see where we are."

Roger made his way out to the desk, got the appointment wallet and a schedule for the next day, including an appointment with somebody over in the Medical Sciences lab building. Then he went back down to Desk C. The receptionist there presented him with an enormous plastic jug and funnel in one paper bag and a small wide-mouth plastic jar with a screw cap in another paper bag.

"I've got to carry these things with me everywhere I go?" Roger asked.

"Everywhere," the woman said.

"I'll look like an ass," Roger said.

"Nobody notices it in Rochester," the receptionist said with a cheery smile. "After all, that's why people are here."

He departed with his jugs, feeling like Marley dragging his chain along behind him. In his room he read the instructions that came with each jug, sighed and poured himself a large bourbon. He telephoned for a dinner reservation at Michael's, three or four blocks from the hotel, and then had another couple of drinks before preparing to go. No date tonight in Rochester, he reflected. Unless he decided to go pub-crawling. *With a plastic jug in each hand? Ridiculous.* It occurred to him suddenly that there might not be going to be any dates in Rochester, period, if today's experience was any indication. *They're all either married or frigid*, he thought gloomily. *Well, maybe there's a singles bar or a topless bar with some kind of action.* After a final drink he set the two jugs down on the floor and went in to shower and shave. He dressed in the casual-sincere fashion befitting a young man on the town, discarded a tie and wore his shirt open with a bead choker. Then he looked down at the jugs on the floor. "I'll be damned if I'm going to carry those things all over Rochester just in case I have to go to the john," he said to himself. "I'll be goddamned if I will." He left the jugs on the floor, locked his room and started down the corridor toward the elevator. There he found two dignified older gentlemen obviously going out to dinner, waiting with their wives for the elevator to come. Each of them had a jug in a large paper bag along with him. Muttering under his breath, Roger went back to his room, retrieved his two jugs and started off for the restaurant with one in each hand.

"I'm afraid," the thin man said across the coffee table, "that I may not be able to enlighten you too much about what keeps this institution running. It's not a matter of secrecy or anything like that. I'm just not sure that anybody knows. Mayo Clinic is simply unlike any other medical organization in the world. I guess it always has been."

The speaker was Dr. John Bagley, a tall, thin rheumatologist who'd been on the Clinic staff for fifteen years. When I had asked for information about the auxiliary personnel of the Clinic—the nurses, aides, receptionists, clerks, technicians and so forth—I was referred to him as chairman of the Personnel Committee. Now, with his office schedule completed this Wednesday evening, we sat in the Kahler coffeeshop sipping iced tea and shivering from the effects of an all-too-efficient air-conditioning system after the 100° heat outside.

"What you're saying," I said, "is that there isn't any expert on Mayo personnel."

"Right," Bagley said. "But I'll tell you whatever I can."

"One thing is obvious," I said. "When you put them all together, there are a whole lot of Mayo personnel."

He nodded. "Over five thousand Clinic employees, give or take a couple hundred, plus another five thousand in the two hospitals. Ten thousand in all. And about eighty percent of them are women. It's that kind of operation. If you're running a steel mill, you hire men. When you need clerks and aides and receptionists and technicians, you hire women."

"I've also noticed that none of them ever seems to stand still. It's absolutely amazing. Everybody seems to be working like mad all the time. I went walking through that accounting department the other day, and over through some of the labs, and hardly anybody even looked up. In fact, Mr. See stopped by a couple of the girls checking bills on the computers and talked about what they were doing, right over their shoulders, and they paid no attention whatever."

Dr. Bagley nodded. "I believe it," he said. "In fact, it's one major reason we can offer top-quality medical services here and still keep our fees very modest compared to other institutions. These girls here really *work*." He looked up at me. "You've seen how other medical institutions operate. You know how often you see personnel sitting around talking, drinking coffee, dropping their work on the floor and forgetting to pick it up, laughing and joking and flirting with the guy across the way, or just sitting on their thumbs, coming in late and leaving early? Why, if those places get two hours of honest work out of their people in the course of an eight-hour day, they're *lucky*. But they pay for eight hours, all the same, you can bet your boots. We don't have that problem here. These girls do eight honest hours' work for eight hours' pay. And believe me, that's getting to be damned near unheard of in this country any more."

"So what's the magic here?" I asked. "Do you have so many applicants that these girls are all scared for their jobs?"

"They're not scared. And we don't have that many applicants, either. In fact, we're constantly recruiting new people to cover the dropouts—the girls who leave and go elsewhere—but that's not because of the job." He shook his head. "Actually the difference is the particular quality of the people who work here. It's as simple as that."

I studied Dr. Bagley's face, trying to figure out what, exactly, he was trying to tell me. "Well," I said cautiously, "I must say I haven't seen any minority-group employees around here to speak of."

Bagley laughed. "You think we're purposely squeezing them out? Discriminatory hiring practices and all that? You couldn't be farther off target. You just show us some minority-group applicants that we can put to work and we'll hire them every time. It'd help our image, if nothing else. But where are we going to find these minority-group applicants? Minnesota has one of the lowest percentages of black people of any state in the union, and ninety-nine point five percent of them live and work in the Twin Cities. Why would they want to come down here to a small, traditionally white community with no black support, no black subculture, no black nothing? Indians, you say? They're scattered throughout the state a bit more, but most of them are still in the northern half. And many just aren't qualified to handle the kind of work we need done. Chicanos? What Chicanos? This is nowhere near the Southwest, and it's never been a big state for migrant workers. There may be ten Chicanos in the whole state of Minnesota, and three of them already work here."

Bagley paused to sip at his tea. "The truth is almost embarrassing when you state it bluntly, but here it is: These girls working for us are virtually all of them God-fearing white Anglo-Saxon Protestant women who've had the old Middle American work ethic beaten into their heads since the day they were born, and when they're hired to work here they figure that means *work*. Most of them are farm girls from the country nearby. They come from families where the day's work starts hours before dawn and doesn't end until dark, and they've been washing and polishing and scrubbing floors and doing dishes and feeding the chickens and slopping the hogs since they were five years old. Coming down to work at Mayo's is a lead-pipe cinch for them; hell, a good busy eight-hour shift of work here may be the first real rest they've ever had in their lives."

"And I suppose you pay good wages?" I asked.

"Oh, yes. Entirely equitable wages. And all the fringe benefits, and so forth. We're not exploiting anybody."

"It sounds as if you have the best of all possible worlds here, as far as your personnel are concerned."

"Yeah," Dr. Bagley said glumly. "I suppose so."

"Then why the high turnover rate you spoke about? Are there some other problems?"

The doctor nodded. "Men," he said.

"*Men?* Well, I can see that you might have a regular wolf pack around here—"

"No, no, no, it isn't that. It *really* isn't that. The problem is *lack* of men. Rochester, Minnesota, has got to be the most female-overloaded small city in the entire United States. The girls don't leave because they hate their jobs. They leave because there aren't any eligible men around. These girls are out on the Kalahari Desert without a water bottle."

"No men? With all the people wandering through here week after week?" I said.

"Well, but those are patients."

"Ah. You mean there's some policy that the girls can't date patients?"

The doctor squeezed lemon in his tea and sighed. "Not really," he said. "Not as a matter of formal policy. When the girls are off duty, they can do anything they feel like doing. But it doesn't make sense for them, dating patients. For one thing, the male patients who are young enough to be attractive aren't here for fun and games, generally speaking. They're here because they're sick. They've got problems. The girls don't know how sick they may be, or what problems they may have, but they know they wouldn't be here if they didn't have them. For another thing, even when the male patients are reasonably young and attractive and look halfway plausible, nine out of ten of them are married. They're only here for a few days before they go back home to Kansas City. Now look at it from the girls' point of view: What does this offer *them?* Most of these girls are strongly family-oriented. Many are quite religious and completely out of touch with the swinging life in the big cities. They aren't remotely interested in sleeping around. They're looking for good, solid husbands and homes and families, whereas the attractive male patients who come here, if they're looking for anything at all, are looking for a quick lay. The girls get trapped once or twice, get burned once or twice, and they start asking themselves, 'Who needs *this?*' And they're right. All these guys are going to give them is a good case of North African gonorrhea—or ten years' worth of genital herpes—and the word gets around pretty fast that the smart girl doesn't mess around dating patients."

Bagley spread his hands. "On top of that, lots of these girls go home to the farm on weekends. Lots of them have six-foot-two, two-hundred-and-twenty-pound farmhand boyfriends back home, and let me tell you, those boys on the farm are not what you would call sexually liberated. And finally—" the doctor took another sip from his glass—"these girls *do* know what is probably an unwritten rule around here—to wit, that if one of them gets into some big messy scandal with a patient, with lots of bad publicity, she's going to be discharged so fast she won't know what hit her. Now when you add all those things together, you begin to see why the whole idea of dating patients seems pretty ridiculous to the girls."

"But what about really *eligible* men?" I said.

"They don't stay eligible very long around here. Let me tell you something. A few years ago IBM wanted to build a big computer facility in Rochester with five thousand employees, mostly male. Well, the town burghers were delighted to have a second industry around this place—but the first thing they asked was: 'How many *unmarried* men?' It worked out pretty well, too. The IBM facility is out there to the west of town, going strong, and a lot more of our girls nowadays seem to be married. But there are still plenty of them moving on to greener fields all the time."

We flagged a waitress to refill our glasses as I mulled over what Dr. Bagley had said. "One other thing puzzles me," I said. "I see girls in white all over the place, but precious few have nurses' caps and precious few have RN on their name tags. Where do you hide all the nurses?"

"We don't really have very many in the Clinic," Dr. Bagley said. "In the hospitals, yes, but not in the Clinic. We don't need them there."

"I thought *every* doctor had his office nurse, or at least shared one," I said.

"It's just unnecessary for us," Bagley said. "Look, we have everything we need in our office examining rooms. A few necessary examining instruments, a few necessary reagents, a stand with alcohol sponges and the sterile needles and the Bard-Parker blades, et cetera. We need someone to show the patients in, but an aide can do that. And we're deliberately organized not to need a nurse during our examinations, at least on the medical floors."

"What about things like pelvic exams?"

"When the time comes for the pelvic exam, we do it," Dr. Bagley said. "Everything we need is there to take Pap smears. We have disposable, prelubricated plastic vaginal specula—who needs a nurse?"

"Don't you, as a witness, so the patient doesn't start screaming rape?" I said.

Bagley laughed. "Yes, of course every doctor's heard that moldy old scare story. But have you ever stopped to think how much money the 'protection' of having a nurse present would cost the patient out of *her* pocket? We just haven't bothered with that 'nurse-witness' rubbish for decades, and *never once* have we been bothered by a lawsuit. Not once. Now, down on the surgical floors where they actually *need* nurses as assistants for minor surgery, that's something else—but even there, generally, the residents and Fellows act as the first assistants, so they don't need so many nurses either. It isn't a matter of cheapness—it's just a matter of common sense and keeping the patient's bill as low as possible."

At this point I heard a beeping sound and Dr. Bagley started. "Better find a phone," he said. "I'll be back in a moment." He disappeared in the direction of the phone booths and was back two minutes later, looking apologetic. "A patient at Methodist that I have to go see," he said. "But if there's anything else you'd like to know, maybe we can meet later?" He deftly picked up the tab just as I was reaching for it and smiled. "At least," he said, "maybe this gives you some insight into how the place operates."

Mildred Hulbert's reunion with Tim MacMichael and his family the previous evening had been thoroughly pleasant. Mary MacMichael had vetoed dinner out and had prepared a ham and potato salad picnic supper to be eaten in their pleasant green back yard shaded by two huge spreading oak trees. Tim had been only a few minutes late home from the Clinic. Next morning he prepared breakfast for Millie and himself without disturbing the others. "We'll drive over to the office together," he said. "I arranged a first-morning appointment for you to see Jerry Whitehead. He's a fine young surgeon, came out here from Massachusetts General in Boston to join us about five years ago. I think you'll like him."

As they drove through the quiet morning streets toward the big gray building Millie said, "Tim, does this sort of thing *always* have to mean surgery? I mean, like a radical mastectomy?"

The man looked over his half-glasses at her. "The answer to the first question is probably yes—a lump in the breast usually means surgery of some sort. What kind of surgery is something else." He looked back at the road, stopped for a stop sign. "Obviously Jerry will need to examine you, see what kind of a lump it is and where and make sure you're in good shape otherwise. I'm sure he'll want mammograms— that's breast X-rays—and probably ultrasound studies too. He'll probably have you see an oncologist, too, down in the Curie Pavilion."

"Oncologist?"

"Fancy word for cancer specialist."

Millie sniffed. "You doctors and your fancy words," she said. "Oncology repeats phylogeny—they taught me that in grade school and I still don't know what it means. Or was it ontogeny?"

MacMichael glanced over to see if Millie was pulling his leg, decided that she was and went on. "Anyway, after all that, Jerry will put all the pieces together and recommend what he thinks is the best way to go. I might say I have the greatest possible confidence in that man. He did Ada's surgery last Thanksgiving, just a simple mastectomy, as I know she's told you, and she's had no problem of any sort since. I think you can count on him to help you make the best decision."

As a matter of fact, Millie *didn't* particularly like Jerry Whitehead at first. He seemed so *terribly* young (but then what doctors didn't, these days, to an eighty-year-old woman?) and terribly precise and scientific, with none of the comfortable old-shoe easygoing manner of a man like Tim

MacMichael and none of the impression of intense personal concern that older doctors somehow manage to project whether they really feel it or not. He wore one of those silly hair-dos the young men went for these days, all coiffed so prettily around his ears, with a sport jacket and slacks that seemed awfully loud—the sort of outfit her husband wouldn't have been seen dead in, Millie reflected.

On the other hand, the young surgeon seemed totally unhurried as he took her history and reviewed her Clinic chart from previous visits, and he had a gentle touch as he examined her. When he finished his examination he said, "Mrs. Hulbert, there certainly is a lump in that breast that we have to investigate further. What's more, with this sort of situation, we like to move as quickly as possible. So I'm going to plan a busy day for you. The girl at the desk will give you a list of appointments starting in about half an hour. You should be all finished by four with plenty of time for lunch, so I'd like to see you here again at four o'clock."

"You mean today?"

"Today. We'll go over everything together at that time."

It *was* a busy day, starting with X-rays of her chest as well as the mammograms she had expected. Early on she was given an injection of a radioactive isotope and returned several hours later to radiology to have a bone scan—an exam she had never heard of and, to her intense irritation, no one would explain to her. At another laboratory two other forms of breast examination were performed, one in which a metal rod was touched to her breasts, immediately casting shadows on a television screen, the other involving a darkened room and a lamp that somehow resembled a very dull red electric heater. Blood was drawn and urine was collected. Other studies were done, and she spent about half an hour with the oncologist, who repeated Dr. Whitehead's exam but refused to tell her anything of what he thought.

By the time Millie Hulbert was back at Dr. Whitehead's office at four o'clock (without lunch because she'd been too upset to want to eat) she was tired and snappish. She was also extremely apprehensive. The chair in the West-6 waiting room was uncomfortable and the arthritis in her hip was kicking up a storm. She tried to leaf through a paperback book she had picked up at the newsstand down in the subway, her invariable way of passing a bit of time, but couldn't even seem to get her glasses to focus. She waited twenty minutes, thirty, then fifteen minutes more. She was about to say "Oh piffle" and leave when her name was finally called, and a few moments later Dr. Whitehead rejoined her in the same room in which they had met early in the morning.

"I'm sorry to hold you up," he said. "We're always running late at this time of day and I had some trouble getting your blood-study reports. I also wanted to talk to Dr. Grossman in the Radiology Department in person about your mammograms and bone scan."

"Well, I hope they showed something," Millie snapped. "Or else I hope they didn't. I don't know which."

Dr. Whitehead leaned back in his chair. "Well, here is the situation," he said. "The mammograns did show something, confirmed by the ultrasound but not picked up by the infrared studies. The mass is in all probability a tumor; some bits of calcium showed up in the area, and that's a very significant finding."

"Of cancer?"

The doctor nodded. "Right," he said. "It appears very small and very early, which is all in your favor."

"So what were all those bone-scan things? And all the blood tests?"

"Frankly, I was more than a little bit worried about that mole that you had removed five years ago," the surgeon said. "We know that was a malignant melanoma, and we know that kind of cancer sometimes recurs quickly in widespread places. We wanted to rule that out as a factor, if possible, before doing a biopsy on this breast lump. At this point I'm ninety-nine percent satisfied that we're dealing with a breast tumor that has nothing to do with the other thing at all."

Millie gripped the arm of the couch. "At least *that's* something," she said. "So what do we do about this?"

"I think we should remove it as quickly as possible."

"You mean a radical mastectomy?"

"Well, I don't really think that's going to be necessary,"

Dr. Whitehead said. "In fact, I think something far less extensive is in order." He hitched around in his chair. "If you were a much younger woman, maybe in your forties, and there was no evidence to convince us that this lump was probably malignant, we would probably simply biopsy the lump right here in the office, then wait for a pathology report and plan our next move from there. However, you're not in your forties, and I'm at least seventy-five percent sure that this is a malignancy. Therefore, I think we should have you in the hospital for the procedure. First we'll biopsy the lump and have a preliminary pathologist's report right while you're there in the operating room under anesthesia. If the report is negative, we're home free—although once in a rare while the later, final pathologist's report does find malignant cells. If the report is positive, then I think we should take a wider bit of tissue around where the mass was and at the same time explore the axilla—the area up under the arm—to remove the lymph nodes to which this kind of tumor might spread first. This would really amount to taking a wedge or segment of breast tissue, like a small slice of pie, with a fairly small incision, very little breast deformity and no problem of arm-swelling and so forth. In short, in your particular case I think we should do the very least we can get away with doing and still be as sure as we can of getting rid of the cancer."

Suddenly she found herself viewing Dr. Whitehead in an entirely different light. "Does Tim MacMichael know about this?" she asked.

He nodded. "I discussed it with him at some length about a half an hour ago. He'll drop by to see you in the hospital this evening and so will some of my surgical team. I've already reserved your room. You'll have to be over there for check-in by six o'clock, so you'd better hustle now or you'll miss your supper."

"That's at St. Mary's?"

"At Methodist. Just across the street past the Curie Pavilion. Tim said he'd bring your toothbrush when he comes. That's all you'll need."

She took the elevator down to the lobby, stepped out into the hot late-afternoon sun. She'd known it was going to be something like this the minute she found the miserable thing, but now instead of apprehension she felt relief. At least they seemed to know exactly what to do about it here—and at this point it didn't sound nearly as dreadful as she had imagined it would.

In a pleasant suburb of Fargo, North Dakota, Jake Petri watched a china teacup slip out of his fingers and shatter on the kitchen floor. His wife let out a cry. "Oh, Jake," she said, "that was one of Mother's best cups and they're so fragile—" She stopped suddenly, looking at her husband.

Jake set the dish towel aside and bent over to pick up the pieces. Halfway down he stood up again abruptly, shaking his head. "I'm sorry, you're going to have to do it," he said and walked out into the living room to sit down.

Mary Petri followed him. "Jake, is it the same old thing again?"

"The same old thing."

"But Dr. Johnson's medicine—"

"It's not helping." Jake looked up at his wife. "I can't put up with this any more, kid. This right arm gets so numb I can't hold onto anything, or write a note, or even dial a phone. At the office I can't get the words to come straight half the time when I'm dictating. I can't even organize a brief in my mind any more. I haven't got a quarter of the strength I used to have, and lately something's been funny with my vision too. Dr. Johnson says it's probably just nerves, but I don't believe him. I'm going to get Johnny to fly me down to Rochester tomorrow."

Mary Petri said nothing—Jake was not a man to take suggestion too well—but now that he'd said it, she was vastly relieved. She didn't know what was going on with this man she loved so much, but she knew for certain it was not "just nerves." Eight months before, at the age of sixty-three, Giacomo Petri had been an active, robust man, apparently in the flower of good health. Years before, when he was a sharp and energetic young lawyer, he had come to Fargo for reasons long since forgotten and opened a law practice. A small, physically powerful and darkly handsome young man in those days, he had fought the long silent battle of the Italian-American scrapping to gain a foothold in a closed, rigid, Midwestern community with only a handful of Catholics of Mediterranean origin to back him up. It had seemed an endless struggle, but bit by bit Jake Petri had won it. He was a good lawyer. He worked like a plow horse, eighteen hours a day. He got results for his clients. People could always reach him, no matter what day or hour, no matter how niggling the problem.

After a while he became established and then, very slowly, prosperous. As he reached his middle years and began graying handsomely, more and more of the really lucrative legal work began coming his way, things that people didn't want to trust to some young wise guy just out of law school—the estate probates, the trust papers, the complex business contracts and the local corporate tax work. Thus at fifty or so his income was still rising each year; the children were gone by then, tuitions all provided for; they had their own comfortable retirement fund in securities; and Jake and Mary were both beginning to say maybe he should slow down, not work so hard, maybe they should do some traveling, take that trip back to Italy they'd never quite managed. Of course Jake knew in his heart of hearts that he wasn't going to slow down, that hard work was as much a part of his nature as breathing—but still it was fun to think and talk about it, maybe even make some plans.

Then one day eight months ago, sitting at his desk in his office, Jake had reached for his pen and dropped it on the floor three times before he could get hold of it. He felt suddenly dizzy, almost sick to his stomach, and his vision seemed blurry for a few moments, with two images instead of one. When the episode passed, as it did after an hour or so, he noticed an odd sort of numbness in the thumb and forefinger of his right hand, and it was still there the next day. He marked it all down to a little arthritis; he'd been having twinges in his joints recently, though otherwise he felt fine—until the same thing happened again ten days later.

He didn't mention it to Mary—she would only worry—but he did go to see Dr. Johnson, a superannuated old family doctor of eighty-three who checked him over after a fashion and clapped him on the back and declared him sound as a dollar. "It's probably nothing, Jake. You've just been working too hard, that's all. Why not take a week off? Do some work in the garden."

It was two months before anything else happened, and then it was much the same except that this time his tongue wouldn't work right either. He was dictating a letter and began to hear his words coming out in a slur, as if he were three sheets to the wind, except that Jake rarely drank anything but a little red wine. This too seemed to pass quickly, but the interval between recurring episodes grew shorter. When he saw Dr. Johnson next the old man was impressed enough at least to prescribe some pills. Jake glanced at the prescription and said, "But that's just aspirin."

"Very good drug," Dr. Johnson said. "Kind of thins the blood on us old guys. But if you don't think that's strong enough, I'll give you another one too. These little red pills will fix you up."

Jake went home, looked at the pills, said something vulgar in Italian and dumped them into the toilet.

That night he told Mary about the problem. He knew it would make her begin to hover and fret, but he himself was beginning to worry. The numbness in the hand and arm had gotten progressively worse and didn't seem to recover. His vision was off a great deal now, and his whole level of energy seemed reduced; some mornings he could hardly get out of bed and was leaning more and more heavily on the girls at the office to handle paper preparation that he had always done himself. Then one day in a magazine he read an article about TIAs, or transient ischemic attacks—so-called "little strokes" that came and went but that some of the medical hotshots thought were warnings of a major stroke to come. The article told how new diagnostic tests could sometimes pin down where the trouble was coming from, and sometimes surgery on the blood vessels in the head could prevent a bad one before it had time to happen. The article, written by a doctor, called it "the most delicate operation in the world" and warned that even just the diagnostic studies alone could be fatal—yet, when the operation worked, lives could be saved that might otherwise be lost.

Several big medical centers were listed where experts did this kind of work. One of the places mentioned was the Mayo Clinic.

His decision finally made, Jake didn't waste time. He talked to the pilot of the local charter plane service and arranged for an early-morning flight to Rochester. Then he called his junior law partner and told him he was taking a few days off, never mind why. As they undressed for bed that night Mary said, "I think you're smart, Jake. I'm glad you're going to get to the bottom of this."

"Aw, it's probably going to turn out to be nothing," Jake said. "Probably just nerves, like old Doc Johnson said. But we gotta spread the wealth a little, keep those docs down there in pizza. Otherwise they might just starve out."

Jake Petri didn't realize yet that he had been living the last eight months with one foot in the grave and the other on a banana peel.

7

Rochester, Minnesota / *1883–1893*

The story goes that Will and Charlie Mayo declared more than once that the smartest thing they ever did was to pick the right parents. There was probably more truth than fiction to that. They also liked to say their success was primarily due to choosing the right time and place to be born, and there was truth to that also. Certainly they were children of the times, and the times were absolutely providential for young men who fiercely wanted to become surgeons.

Throughout their lives the Mayo boys had grown up in a family deeply immersed in medicine, their father already doing pioneering surgery in back-country America. As the boys approached maturity, each in his turn was sent away for the finest medical education available in the country at the time, however lacking such education may have been. Upon completion of their formal medical training—two or three years in those days—they had a built-in and thriving general practice of medicine and surgery waiting for them back home. (By the early 1880s the elder Dr. Mayo had one of the three largest medical practices south of the Twin Cities and perhaps the single largest practice in all of southern Minnesota.)

But more important to their future than a ready-made practice to come home to was the fact that the great debate about Listerism was raging hot and heavy at the precise time that the Mayo brothers were in medical school. The whole revolutionary concept of surgery as a serious approach to medical treatment was beginning to blossom, just waiting for a pair of bright and aggressive young men from the Midwest to come along and make it their own.

Joseph Lister's great discovery—that bacteria-killing carbolic acid applied to clean open wounds could help prevent surgical infection—was soon proven in his own operating room. But Lister was an intensely practical and logical man. Clearly there were bacteria all over the patient's skin: Pasteur had demonstrated that. Logically, there had to be bacteria everywhere else also—on the surgeon's hands, on his clothing, on the garments of his assistants, in the coughs and sneezes of people in the operating room, in the very air of the place. If cleaning the open wound with carbolic acid helped reduce infection, then it followed that destroying bacteria everywhere else possible around the surgical patient would reduce chances of infection even more.

This meant to Lister that he had to keep not only the wound itself clean but everything else in the operating room as well—not just aesthetically clean but *antiseptically* clean, germ-killingly clean. Maybe he couldn't destroy *all* bacteria that might contact the patient, but he could destroy a lot of them. To do this, Lister began spraying the air of the operating room with carbolic acid solution just before an operation. He scrubbed his hands in carbolic acid solution, and so did everyone else present. He used the antiseptic to scrub the instruments, to soak down the sponges and dressings and to paint the patient's skin where the incision was to be made. Everything that touched or came near the patient had to be antiseptically clean, so that Lister performed his operations in the midst of an eye-burning fog of carbolic acid solution, with great pails and buckets of the stuff around for handwashing and dressing-dipping, and he and everyone else emerged sopping wet and reeking after an operation.

The results of all this bother? In Joseph Lister's operating room the rate of wound infections among his patients dropped precipitously. It was not just a *little* change; it was downright unbelievable. High percentages of post-surgical patients were healing swiftly without infection who would once have died for sure, or at the very least would have suffered long, drawn-out septic wound infections with recovery dragging on for months or even years. In 1867 Lister described his "antiseptic method" of surgery in great detail in a medical paper, one of the great classical dissertations in all medical history. Surgeons in England and Europe opposed him at first—but those who visited his surgery, observed his "antiseptic method" in use and then saw the results he got wiped carbolic acid tears out of their eyes and went home and did likewise.

By 1875 Lister's "antiseptic method" for surgery was widely accepted in the major medical centers of Europe; by 1879 he was being widely celebrated for his life-saving discovery. It was said at the time that his pioneering work would soon have saved more lives than all the wars in history had thrown away. Yet in 1883, when Will Mayo was about to graduate from Michigan Medical College and Charlie was about to enter the Chicago Medical College at Northwestern University, American medical students were *still* not being taught Lister's methods and principles.

Just *why* this was true is hard to understand today. Of course news traveled slowly in those days—but surgeons were constantly going to Europe to study, and the word of Lister's work had reached America decades before. And in fact, there *were* a few surgeons in America in the early 1880s following Lister's practices and obtaining Lister's results. There were just a great many more who weren't and flatly refused to bother, results or no results.

Doubtless one reason was that the whole business was a bloody bother. Hours had to be spent just preparing the operating room—scrubbing down the table, soaking sponges and instruments in antiseptic, mopping down floors and walls, filling basins and atomizers full of solution and so on. Once the operation began, someone had to go around spraying the air, the patient, the surgeons and everything else throughout the procedure. And then when the operation was over, there was this enormous mess to clean up and the whole procedure had to be repeated before the next operation could begin.

Those doughty surgeons who were *really convinced* that all this folderol did some good were willing to go through with it. But there were still many surgeons, for example, who *simply didn't believe in bacteria*. Others thought maybe Lister's techniques were necessary in the "bad air" of old city hospitals but weren't needed in places with "good air." Some surgeons kept forgetting that once they washed their hands in the carbolic acid they had to *keep* them clean. If they scratched their hair or bent over to pick up a dropped instrument, they had to go scrub their hands all over again, and this quickly got to be a bore. Some surgeons tried halfway measures, making gestures toward antisepsis without really achieving it and then, when their infection rate remained just as high as ever, would say, "See? All this business is just hokum." Finally, not a few surgeons tried the carbolic acid spray in their operating rooms and found the stuff made them ill.

As it was, Michigan Medical School at Ann Arbor at the time Will Mayo was attending, for all its other good qualities, was making little effort to teach antiseptic surgical techniques. Some of Will's major surgical instructors wanted nothing to do with it. Thus when Will James Mayo graduated from Michigan and received his M.D. degree on June 28, 1883, he probably had only the most nodding acquaintance with the one vital revolutionary principle that was later destined to provide him his own great opportunity as a surgeon.

With Charles Mayo at Chicago Medical College the story was a little different, fortunately. Will was already back home practicing with their father when Charlie entered Chicago in the fall of 1885. With merely average grades, Charlie was no leader of his class; indeed, one of the lowest grades he received was in a course on Principles and Practices of Surgery! However, most of the surgeons at Chicago were converts to Listerism, and Charlie obtained a solid background in antiseptic technique. He also observed something else just appearing on the surgical scene: the presence of trained nurses in the Chicago hospitals, some of whom were already beginning to specialize in antiseptic operating-room procedures—a factor that gave Listerism an enormous boost. Charlie, however, would not be taking this expertise in antiseptic surgery back to Rochester and putting it into practice until his graduation from Chicago Medical School in 1888.

In Rochester, meanwhile, Will Mayo, at the age of twenty-two, had already set his sights on surgery, and they were set high. Many people back home imagined that the older doctor and his son would never manage together as far as surgery was concerned, since the old man was enamored of surgery too. Some even imagined that this young twenty-two-year-old would move on to a surgical practice in St. Paul or Chicago after a couple of years in his father's office. But nothing was farther from Will Mayo's mind. "I expect," he told amused inquirers, "to remain in Rochester and become the greatest surgeon in the world." At the time, the remark must have sounded silly and certainly arrogant. Ten years later it didn't sound either silly or arrogant.

The truth was that father and son worked well together, for the practice was busy and there was plenty for both of them to do. This was a time, in the mid-1880s, when many wagon trains were passing through southern Minnesota on their way to the Dakota Territory—immigrants in such numbers that two Dakota states were to be admitted to the Union in 1889. The Mayos' name and reputation had become famous enough by then that many of these people going through, some as far as Wyoming, remembered and came back when they had illnesses to be treated. They also told their neighbors in the Territory about the Mayos, so that more and more out-of-town patients began coming to Rochester to see the two doctors. Usually these were patients with serious, long-standing illnesses, often surgical illnesses.

There was, of course, no hospital in Rochester at all in those days, so these out-of-town visitors had to take hotel rooms. Fortunately a certain Mrs. Carpenter in Rochester had a large house which she converted into a nursing home capable of accommodating eight or ten patients. Here the two Mayos did their surgery, using an operating table and other equipment that they could wheel from room to room as necessary. Even without benefit of antiseptic techniques their surgical results, in terms of recoveries and deaths, compared very favorably with the big medical centers—which was to say, they were astoundingly good for Minnesota. More and more, these operations became regular medical meetings, with doctors from all the surrounding communities coming to watch their major operations.

In modern-day terms, of course, their results were not so splendid. During the decade of the 1880s the older doctor did a total of thirty-six ovariectomies; twenty-seven of those patients recovered, but nine died. In much of the surgery that father and son were undertaking, they were literally "learning by doing"—making things up as they went along, without much instruction, nor even a very clear idea of what was surgically possible and what was not in a given case. Nor was there really any way that young Will could obtain any formal surgical instruction to supplement the basic medical training he'd received at Michigan. There was no such thing as graduate study in medicine at the time, nor any systematic, organized training in surgery. In fact, the only thing Will could do was precisely what his father had done before him: go to the place where the best surgery in the country was being performed and watch it being done. As early as 1884, before Charlie had even gone off to medical school, Will Mayo made the first of a long series of such educational trips and encountered a surgical disease that was to bring him his earliest surgical fame.

This trip was to the New York Polyclinic to observe the work of one Dr. Henry B. Sands. The arrangements were very simple. No applications were made, no letters of introduction written. Young Will Mayo simply traveled to New York, prepared to spend six weeks or so and appeared early in the morning at the operating room of the surgeon he wanted to observe. Sometimes the surgeon would treat such an uninvited guest kindly and sometimes he would not, but the "big surgeons," whether kindly disposed or ill-tempered, all seemed to share one quality in common: They loved to be watched. Will Mayo spent six weeks watching Dr. Sands, who was trying to treat a mysterious surgical illness known as "perityphlitic abscess" with rather indifferent success.

This condition had been baffling surgeons for decades; no one knew for sure just what it was or why it happened. Typically the patient—often a relatively young person in bounding good health—would suddenly have an episode of severe indigestion, abdominal pain, a little fever and a little vomiting. This disorder would seem to get worse for a period of forty-eight hours or so, sometimes longer, and then would improve, rather abruptly, quite of its own accord. The trouble, however, was not over. A great many of these patients suddenly collapsed and died within a day or so after their reprieve and were found at autopsy to have extensive peritonitis. Others went into a period of prolonged chronic illness, with spiking fevers, continuing lower abdominal pain, weight loss, nausea, vomiting and general physical decline. Of course in those days, considering the high rate of death from infection following abdominal surgery, neither patient nor surgeon was eager to have the abdomen opened to find out what the problem was, but when finally forced to, the surgeon would find a huge abscess in the lower right-hand corner of the abdomen. If that abscess could be drained and if the patient did not subsequently die of peritonitis or wound infection from the surgery, he might make it back to health after a long and tedious convalescence.

The disease, of course, was what we know today as common appendicitis. The initial symptoms arose from an attack of acute appendicitis as we know it today, in which the appendix becomes inflamed, then actively infected and finally gangrenous. The "reprieve" of symptoms occurred when the gangrenous appendix ruptured, and between thirty and forty percent of patients died during the next seventy-two hours from generalized peritonitis. Those who survived that blow, or were lucky enough to wall off the ruptured appendix and confine the infection to one area of the right lower abdomen, would proceed to form the "perityphlitic abscess." By the time the surgeon finally felt driven to open the abdomen to treat this condition, the patient was already half dead, exceedingly toxic from the continuing infectious process going on in his body; these abscesses could become the size of a football by the time the surgeon got to them. Even then, just draining such an abscess carried a frightening mortality rate. The surgeon would simply go to the patient in his hospital bed, give him a little chloroform and thrust a scalpel through the abdominal wall into the abscess without further ceremony, allowing liters of pus to drain out of the wound then and there. It was small wonder so many of them died.

With Dr. Henry Sands at the New York Polyclinic, Will Mayo encountered a different way of thinking about treating this illness. A few surgeons were gradually beginning to see a consistent pattern in the natural history of the illness. Here, it seemed to them, was a small localized infection that began in the appendix, for whatever reason. As long as it remained localized in that organ it wasn't in itself dangerous; it was only when it perforated and spread infection far and wide around the interior of the abdomen that the patient was in grave danger of death. But couldn't the infection be diagnosed while it was still localized in the appendix? If a surgeon could do that, then he might open the patient's abdomen early, at the very beginning of the illness, find the infected appendix before it could rupture and remove it. Certainly such an approach ought to salvage a great many patients who might otherwise die.

And indeed it did. With early diagnosis and early surgery to remove the appendix, there were far fewer deaths from peritonitis, fewer patients who developed the huge abdominal abscesses. Returning home to Rochester, Will Mayo put this idea to work, striving for earlier and earlier diagnosis and surgery on the cases he saw. By 1888 Will had treated twenty or more such cases successfully and felt confident enough in his experience to read a paper about it before an annual meeting of the Minnesota Medical Society. There were startled faces at that meeting, and well there might have been. Here was a young bumpkin from the boondocks of southern Minnesota, barely five years out of medical school, reporting on his experience in one of the most sophisticated and advanced aspects of modern surgery! *His experience!* Yet he was, in fact, one of the first surgeons in the Midwest to perform modern-type appendectomies in any significant numbers.

Soon both brothers were following their father's pattern for learning new surgical techniques and discovering new surgical ideas on a regular basis. They would hear of some bold, innovative or much needed new surgical procedure being pioneered by some surgeon in Washington or Philadelphia or St. Louis or Boston or Chicago. One or the other of the brothers would then go observe the surgeon performing the procedure, make rounds with him on his patients, talk with him, examine the risks and results first hand and try to figure out how the procedure might be done better, or even done at all in Rochester without the benefit of fine city hospital facilities. Then the observer would come home, take what he felt was right about the new procedure, adapt it to the patients he was seeing and begin performing it.

Beyond any doubt these two young Rochester doctors were uncannily sharp observers. They were also incredibly skillful surgeons—skillful enough to be able to refine and improve the new surgical techniques they observed until they were doing better operations than their teachers. And word about the surgery they were doing, and the remarkably good results they were getting, began to spread far beyond the confines of southern Minnesota in the 1880s and 1890s.

Those good results, in large part, were due to the fact that from about 1887 on the Mayo brothers bit the bullet and began practicing consistent and rigid antisepsis in their operating rooms. This one decision alone vastly expanded the scope of surgery that they could undertake. Freed from the specter of wound infection, with ever-growing confidence that they could count on rapid, clean wound healing—and with reliable ether or chloroform anesthesia now available—they were able to perform operations they could not even have dreamed of ten years before. During these two decades of the 1880s and 1890s, for example, Will and Charlie Mayo began performing surgery on the stomach for peptic ulcer disease, intestinal obstruction or cancer. They began doing gall-bladder surgery—not just removing a few stones but removing the whole diseased organ and, later, exploring the common bile duct to dislodge stones that might be impacted there. They did surgery on the thyroid gland to treat thyroid disease, surgery on the eye to remove cataracts, surgery in the pelvis to remove diseased ovaries or surgery to correct badly varicosed leg veins. Not that they were necessarily introducing these procedures for the first time in the area; other surgeons were doing similar operations in the Twin Cities or in isolated areas around the Midwest. But those surgeons were doing one or two cases here and there while the Mayo brothers were doing dozens and dozens and looking around for more.

The one thing they did not have during the early days of their surgery was a hospital, and that was one thing they needed badly. It took an act of providence to provide it.

On August 21, 1883, Rochester was struck by a devastating tornado. Multitudes of people were injured, many more left homeless, and virtually every public house and open space in town was commandeered to take care of them. An order of nuns known as the Sisters of St. Francis, who operated a local convent and school, contributed to the nursing care in one of the temporary hospitals that was set up to meet the emergency. Some time after the crisis was over, Mother Alfred of the Sisters approached old Dr. Mayo with an idea: What would he think if the Sisters were to build a permanent hospital under the sponsorship and direction of the Sisters? At the time (this was while Will was still in medical school and Charlie not yet out of high school) old Dr. Mayo didn't think it was such a good idea, and nothing was done about it. There wasn't really a need for a hospital, he told the Reverend Mother. The place would never support itself. She would probably have a financial disaster on her hands.

Mother Alfred listened and let the idea ride for the moment. Then, after four years of thinking and planning, with financial support from the Roman Catholic Church, she decided to go ahead with her project and asked the old doctor to help her design the hospital. By late 1889 the first unit of

St. Mary's Hospital was built. Old Dr. Mayo was appointed physician-in-charge and his sons had staff appointments. But administrative control of the hospital remained in the hands of the Sisters, first Mother Alfred and then, beginning in 1892, in the hands of a certain Sister Joseph, a singularly gifted administrator who was to hold the position for some forty years.

The new hospital must have seemed a dream come true to the Mayo brothers. Certainly it was a step up from the portable operating facilities of Mrs. Carpenter's nursing home. The new St. Mary's had only a single operating room, but that one was fully equipped by the Mayos from top to bottom, with Charlie Mayo fashioning many of the instruments and, in fact, building his own operating table—a bizarre-looking affair still on view in a St. Mary's Hospital display case today. There were forty-six beds in the hospital, and, in the beginning, the nuns and novices of the order acted as nurses. The rooms were small, furnished with only the barest of necessities: bed, wooden chair, nightstand. True, the place was clumsily located—way out beyond the outskirts of town a mile from the Mayos' downtown office—but that was where the Sisters had been able to buy an inexpensive piece of property, so that was where the hospital was built. Despite this awkwardness, the hospital seemed to have a lot going for it—except for one thing.

That thing would cause little fuss today, but at that time and place it was a major problem and one that ultimately precipitated a fortuitous crisis. The problem was that the hospital was built, owned and administered by Roman Catholics, and Rochester was a fiercely, almost aggressively, Protestant community.

It is hard for us today really to grasp the depth of religious prejudice in this country in the late 1800s, and there were few places where anti-Catholicism was more deeply entrenched than in the Midwest. Old Dr. Mayo and his sons were happy to accept association and staff appointments at the new hospital—but they couldn't get one single other doctor in the community to join the staff. This meant, of course, that the Mayos were the *sole* medical staff of the hospital.

They were also the only doctors in the community admitting patients there. In 1892, when old Dr. Mayo was seventy-three years old, the problem was compounded when Dr. W. A. Allen, a Rochester homeopathic physician, remodeled an old house in downtown Rochester into a hospital of sorts and began operating Riverside Hospital in competition with St. Mary's.

The flash point came when other physicians in town then called upon the Mayos to come to Riverside Hospital and consult with them about patients there. It was a painful decision. The Mayos were not doctors to pass up seeing patients—but ultimately they refused, feeling that they were obligated to give their full support to St. Mary's. Their decision made a lot of people in town angry, but the Mayos simply ignored it and went about their daily rounds. They had done what they thought they should do and that was that. Nor did the town's censure for their affiliation with St. Mary's seem to have much effect on their practice: They were busier than ever. In a short while Riverside Hospital collapsed of its own weight, and the Sisters of St. Francis, in a fine touch of sauce for the gander, established the policy that no patient could be admitted to St. Mary's Hospital who had not first been seen by one of the Mayos. As Helen Clapesattle expressed it in her book *The Doctors Mayo*, "This gave the Mayos in the mid-1890s a curious situation of having a monopoly of the *only* hospital facilities in existence in the whole wide area of southern Minnesota and the *best* hospital facilities in a still wider area."

Indeed, it was a good time and a good situation for the Mayo doctors. They had a thriving practice in a pleasant community. They had good office facilities and—now—good hospital facilities as well. The old man, growing older and less eager to wrestle with lions than he was in his youth, was now relieved in his work by his two sons and could, if he chose, retire at his own pace. The sons were already developing uncommon reputations for their surgical skills—reputations that extended far beyond the boundaries of Rochester. They had patients returning from afar for treatment because they had been treated well by the Mayos previously and thought they were good doctors. Indeed, there were all the elements here of a large, comfortable family medical practice that could keep Will and Charlie Mayo busy for the rest of their lives. In the early 1890s the thought of ever establishing a clinic—*a clinic?*—had never entered their minds.

It was an idea whose time had not yet come.

8

Rochester, Minnesota / *June 1979*

It was ten o'clock in the morning when the little plane Jake Petri had chartered put down at the airfield in Rochester. He and Mary took a cab into town. Mary had known Jake was badly worried when he'd asked her to go with him; Jake was usually a loner when it came to facing crises.

The cab dropped him off in front of the Mayo Building, then took Mary on with their bags to the place they wanted to stay. Not one of the big hotels; Jake's frugal nature rebelled, despite their ample means. "Fancy hotels are for conferences where somebody else is paying the bill," he said. "There are plenty of small motels around." She found one two blocks away from the Mayo Building, clean and comfortable, modest in price, with a kitchenette if she wanted to cook and a small restaurant on the ground floor if she didn't.

At the Clinic Jake went directly to the reception desk. He gave the woman there a brief description of the symptoms he'd been having. The woman listened very carefully until he finished. Then: "All right, Mr. Petri, we'll get working on it. Without an appointment, you'll have to have a priority exam first."

"Can we possibly do that today? I'm getting kind of desperate."

"I understand, and I think we can. Let me just see what we have here." She checked cards in a rack, dialed a four-digit number on the telephone and spoke briefly. "Fine," she said to Jake. "If you can be on West Eight at eleven-thirty, Dr. Teeman will see you. Meanwhile, you *might* just have time to get in on the ten o'clock tour, if you feel like it."

"No, I think I'll just rest," Jake said. "It's been kind of a mean trip." He found a seat in the back of the appointments waiting room, sat down wearily, took off his glasses to wipe his eyes, felt them slip from his fingers to the floor. For a long moment he just looked at them, then shook his head, leaned back in the chair and closed his eyes, leaving the glasses on the floor.

Mary Petri found him there a little while later. "We've got a room at the Clinic View," she said, "with a kitchenette, so I can make a nice supper for you. Now why don't you just doze here, if that's what you feel like doing. I'll go bring you a sandwich or something."

At 11:30 sharp he was on West 8 at the reception desk, and ten minutes later he was called to see the doctor. Dr. Teeman was a very young, very sleepy-looking man who seemed to Jake to be considerably less interested in what he was doing than Jake would have liked. He kept yawning as he started taking a brief, routine-sounding history from Jake—where did he come from (Fargo), had he ever been to Mayo before ("No"), no medical record here? ("No"), and so on and so on in a thoroughly disorganized fashion. The young man kept leaning back in the swivel chair at the desk and closing his eyes, until Jake was afraid he was either going to begin snoring like the dormouse or go over on his head. "Well," Dr. Teeman said from out of his torpor, "there must have been *something* that brought you all the way from Fargo on this particular day. Can you tell me what?"

"Yeah," Jake said. "I think I'm having little strokes."

Young Dr. Teeman sat up in his chair abruptly and looked at Jake Petri. He no longer seemed so sleepy. "I beg your pardon?"

"I said I think I'm having little strokes," Jake said. "I keep dropping things. My right hand is numb, especially the thumb and forefinger. It comes and goes, but never goes completely away. Then there's my vision and my balance—"

"Tell me about dropping things," Dr. Teeman said.

Jake told him. It didn't take long. Jake was an economist with words when he wasn't writing legal briefs, and he knew how to organize his thoughts and express them clearly. He told the doctor about the dizzy spells, the spells of double vision that came and went, the loss of muscular control in his right arm and hand and the steadily increasing numbness that didn't seem to go away; the slowly progressive weariness and loss of energy, the headaches, the loss of appetite and weight loss.

"This double vision," Dr. Teeman said. "Does it last long?"

"Two or three hours. Then once or twice it seemed as if I was looking through a grid of dark lines that made everything look dark."

"And the hand business has been progressive?"

"The numbness. Except that recently I can't really control a pen. And sometimes my tongue doesn't want to work and my thinking gets scrambled. Like something's going wrong with my head."

"That's not so good for a lawyer," Dr. Teeman said.

"Or anybody else."

"This has been going on for eight months?"

"Since it first started, yes. Only at first the spells didn't seem like anything. I was a busy man, I couldn't afford to be sick, and they were easy to ignore. At first."

The young man suddenly pushed his chair back and stood up. "Mr. Petri," he said, "aside from appointment priorities and all that, I want another doctor to see you."

"That's why I'm here," Jake said. "I can come in any time."

"I mean right now. I think we need a really expert opinion. If you don't mind waiting outside there for maybe another hour, I think I can reach the man I want."

Back in the waiting room Jake sat down beside Mary. "He wants another doctor to see me," he said. "It may be a little while. We're supposed to wait."

"I still have that sandwich I brought for you," Mary said.

"No, I couldn't eat it," Jake said. "I've got to get to the bottom of this."

It wasn't an hour's wait after all, more like twenty minutes, when Jake was paged again and returned to Dr. Teeman's examining room. This time Dr. Teeman was accompanied by a much older man, a short little man in his late fifties with sandy graying hair, a florid face and very bright blue eyes. He was introduced as Dr. O'Shaughnessy. "And what kind of doctor are you?" Jake inquired.

"I'm a neurosurgeon," the doctor said, "but don't let that scare you away. I'm also a neurologist, and from the little Dr. Teeman has been able to tell me you might be right that something is going wrong with your head. And if so, we'd better find out what without a whole lot of delay and see if we can do something about it."

The older doctor looked over the history notes Dr. Teeman had written out, then pushed them aside and leaned back in the chair, fixing his sharp blue eyes on Jake Petri. Dr. Teeman remained standing in the corner, and there was no more yawning. Slowly, almost leisurely, as though there were all the time in the world, Dr. O'Shaughnessy went over the ground with Jake that Dr. Teeman had covered—only much, much more. He asked questions that seemed to have no relation to the problem at all. He asked questions Jake Petri couldn't even answer. He asked about Jake's work, about the pressures he was under, about his diet, his drinking, the company he and Mary kept, their political attitudes, their religious affiliations. ("As a good Irishman to a good Italian," Dr. O'Shaughnessy said, "there's a nice Catholic church a block north and a block west of the Clinic building. My family's gone there for years.") For a full three-quarters of an hour Dr. O'Shaughnessy explored the nature of Jake's illness and, it seemed, everything else he could think of to ask about Jake Petri as well. Then he motioned him to the examining table and went through a lengthy and detailed physical examination, murmuring to Dr. Teeman from time to time about his findings.

When at last he had finished and allowed Jake to get dressed, he said, "You say Mary is out there in the reception room? I'd like very much to have her come in here now, if you don't mind. We need to talk about some things I think you both should hear so you can make some decisions."

When Mary was ushered into the room Dr. O'Shaughnessy turned his attention to her. "Mrs. Petri," he said, "your husband has been a strong, healthy man all of his life, and that's good, because it's going to help him now when he needs it. What isn't so good is that I think he's in trouble now, and something is going to have to be done to get him out of it."

"You know what's going on with him?" Mary Petri asked.

"I know several things that *could* be going on with him," the doctor replied. "At this point I don't know which one for sure. The trouble is that none of the things I can think of are very good things to have wrong with you."

"I'd sometimes thought that maybe he was having a stroke," Mary said.

Dr. O'Shaughnessy nodded his head. "Of course you think of that first," he said. "And it's possible that he's already had one, even though I don't think so. Strokes don't usually take place over an eight-month period, and this thing, whatever it is, has been going on progressively for at least that long. Okay, what else could it be? Something growing inside his head could create this picture, some kind of tumor. That's a possibility. A brain tumor could press on nerve centers or blood vessels and cause symptoms like Jake's. So could a brain abscess—a localized infection in the brain tissue that keeps getting bigger and bigger, filling up with pus. Fortunately, we've got some good clean, safe ways to identify things like that if they're there, ways to pinpoint where they are and how big they are. Those same studies could also give us a good idea if there's been a stroke of any magnitude. And those examinations can't do any harm, so we feel pretty free to use them. We'll certainly do them with Jake before considering anything else. But if I had to make a bet right now, I would have to bet that *none* of those things is going on."

"Then what do you think it is?" Jake said.

"I think by far the surest bet is that you're having just what you read about in the magazine—transient ischemic attacks, or TIAs. The word 'ischemic' means 'not enough blood,' and these attacks are brief, passing episodes in which not enough blood is getting to a part of the brain. Now the brain needs a lot of oxygen-rich blood in order to function properly, and when it doesn't get enough blood, even briefly, its function is impaired. Nerve cells can be damaged—nerve cells controlling the vision, controlling the muscles and feeling in the right arm, controlling the tongue, even controlling the ability to think straight. If these periods of blood starvation are very brief, some of the injured nerve cells have a chance to snap back—but maybe others don't, so you have one injury piled on top of another, over and over. This, it seems to me, is what Jake has been sitting here telling me about."

"But why would he have them?" Mary asked. "What causes them?"

"Usually there's some obstruction to blood flow somewhere in the brain. It can be the narrowing of an artery due to spasm, or it can be a partial plugging of an artery with a blood clot. Mostly we're scared of TIAs because so often they turn out to be an early warning of a really massive stroke about to happen, a stroke that can knock out half the body, rob a person of speech or writing, partially paralyze him, maybe even kill him. And once one of those happens, you're in the soup. If you recover at all, it may take months or years and even then it may not be complete. Fortunately, if we can pin down the source of these TIAs and do something to replenish the brain's blood supply, we can sometimes prevent a massive stroke and put an end to the problem for years. Unfortunately, this is the place where you folks first have to make some hard decisions."

"Decisions?" Jake said. "I've already decided I can't go on with this thing the way it is, whatever it is. That's why I'm here. Go ahead, do whatever you have to. Find it and fix it if you can."

"I'm afraid it's not quite that easy," Dr. O'Shaughnessy said.

"Well, I don't have to make any weighty decisions for you to find out if there's some kind of blood-vessel obstruction, do I?" Jake said.

"Unfortunately, I'm afraid you do," Dr. O'Shaughnessy said. "The way we have to go to look for an obstructed blood vessel in the brain is very treacherous. There are real risks

involved—and I don't mean the risk of a little pain or discomfort, or the risk of throwing up after the examination, or
anything like that. In this case, just trying to find out what's
wrong can kill a person—literally."

"What do you have to do?" Jake asked suspiciously.

"One key examination is known as a carotid arteriogram," the doctor said. "This involves threading a thin tube or
catheter from an entry point down in the groin up until the
tip reaches the lower end of the carotid artery—the main
artery supplying blood to the brain. At that point we inject a
dye that's opaque to X rays. We then take a whole series of
rapid-fire X-ray pictures to show where that dye goes to in
the circulatory system of the brain. If there's an obstruction
of some sort—a blockage or narrowing or bulging of a vessel
with a clot in it, for instance—we can *sometimes* see precisely
where it is on those pictures. Not always, but sometimes."

Dr. O'Shaughnessy leaned back in his chair. "Now, if this
sounds to you like a sort of difficult procedure, take my word
for it, it is. It's not any innocuous little thing like a CAT scan.
We have the finest equipment money can buy around this
place, and the people who do the carotid arteriograms are
among the most skillful in the world, with as much or more
experience in what they're doing as anyone else anywhere—
yet we have patients who don't even survive the arteriograms. They die. We have others who come out of it alive but
act as if they'd had a massive stroke. And in fact the procedure can, on rare occasions, *precipitate* a massive stroke,
either right away or up to twenty-four hours later. We have
still other cases where the patient has decided to take this
whopping risk and comes out of it okay, but we don't learn
one single thing from the pictures we've taken, so all the risk
was for nothing. This is why I can't seriously encourage you
to undergo this kind of study until I'm absolutely certain you
clearly understand the risks involved and what they could
mean." He looked from Jake to Mary and back, and he was
not smiling. "I'm not trying to scare you, but you have to
know and understand the truth and I have to know you really
do. Unless I'm personally convinced you both have that understanding and give your consent to the procedure *with* that

understanding, I won't authorize those studies. And if I won't, neither will anyone else in Rochester."

Jake Petri stared at the doctor for a long moment. He'd always respected straight language, and he liked this man—but that wasn't the issue right now. "What are the percentages?" he asked.

"The mortality rate is about one percent for the angiograms alone," Dr. O'Shaughnessy said. "That means that one out of every hundred patients who have that study, on the average, just turn up their toes. The percentage of morbidity—a massive stroke during or following the angiograms, or convulsions, or lasting personality changes—is between ten and fifteen percent. By 'morbidity' we mean morbid results, so to speak—bad results short of death—and that ten to fifteen percent is on top of the one percent mortality. Those are the cold equations you both have to understand."

"But if what you think is going on, I'm going to die from it very soon anyway," Jake said.

The neurosurgeon shook his head. "I don't know that," he said. "I think it's very possible, maybe even probable, but I can't say yes, you'd die. You might go right on and live to be a hundred and seventeen—and believe me, I know some people who very nearly did. I don't think it's very likely, but I can't decide for you on that basis."

"All the same," Jake said, "you're saying that it's your professional opinion that I should go ahead and have this done."

"It's my professional opinion that a procedure exists that can often help doctors like me diagnose and hopefully treat patients like you. There are a number of safe things we can do first to try to pin the diagnosis *without* the angiograms, and it's certainly my professional opinion that we should do those first. It's also my professional opinion that we may well reach a dead end in diagnosing your illness that way, and if we do, I may well be unable to help you without the angiograms. And yes, if the other studies draw a blank, and I know that you fully comprehend the risk involved in the angiograms and could give your truly informed consent to go ahead with them, then it would be my professional opinion that you should have them—but under no other circumstances."

Jake looked at his wife and shrugged. "If what you think is actually going on, I don't stand the chance of an egg on a hot plate. And I think you're telling me the truth about the risk figures, too. So I guess you could say you have your informed consent."

"Well, since we're not backed into a corner this very minute, don't tell me that just yet," Dr. O'Shaughnessy said. "I have some literature about the procedure. I'd like you both to read it tonight. Think about it. Talk it over between you. Also give some thought to what your plans for the future might be, what you might do, if you *did* have an unfortunate result. In the meantime, we have some other things to be done. We need some blood studies, a cardiogram to check on your heart, some chest films to be sure that there isn't something growing in a lung that has spread to your brain—things like that. I'd like to get going with these this afternoon. Then tomorrow we need a CAT scan and some of the other nondangerous studies that I spoke about. We might find we don't need the arteriograms. But meanwhile, you can be thinking and coming to a decision." The doctor stood up in preparation for departing. "Dr. Teeman will get things lined up for this afternoon, but right now I want Jake over in the hospital. Everything can be taken care of from there."

"You really think the hospital's necessary?" Petri asked.

"I really do," the doctor replied. "I don't want to take any chances with you."

"Then tell me one thing," Jake said, stopping the doctor at the door. "Do you think you're really going to be able to do something about this?"

O'Shaughnessy looked startled. "Well, I sure as hell *hope* so," he said. "And you know something?" He looked back and flashed a surprisingly boyish grin at Jake Petri. "I've got a good feeling about you. Between you and me, I think we're going to nail this thing to the wall before we get through."

"But what on earth," I said, *"keeps* them here?"

"Keeps who where?" Art Amundson said, caught off stride.

"Keeps the doctors here in Rochester," I said. "Oh, I don't mean the residents—the ones you call Fellows, the doctors-in-training. They're here at one of the most prestigious medical centers in the world to learn fancy medicine from some of the finest specialists in the world. They can sweat out Rochester for a while—though I bet their wives hate it. And of course your employees have jobs here and this is the part of the country most of them came from anyway, so they're happy enough. But what about the six hundred and eighty-odd staff doctors of Mayo Clinic? What keeps *them* here?"

"Well, it's kind of a nice little town," Art said lamely, obviously offended by the question. "What's wrong with it?"

"Nothing's exactly *wrong* with it," I said. "It certainly is a little town—well, call it a small city, sixty thousand people or so. But what's here? I suppose you have a concert series once a year, an orchestra comes down from the Cities and plays once in a while, and there's a nice public library with extended borrowing privileges. But that's about it. What about theater, ballet, opera? What do these doctors *do?*"

Art shrugged. "I guess they just practice medicine," he said.

"Aw, come on. That's an easy answer, but it doesn't answer anything. There's got to be *some* reason these men come here and stick. Without them you wouldn't have any Mayo Clinic; the place would fall apart overnight."

"That's very true," Art said. "The Mayo Clinic *is* the staff doctors. Everything depends on them—their presence, their expertise, their work, the patients they attract—everything. Without them the other two legs to the footstool—the medical teaching and the medical research—couldn't exist. No, we have to have those doctors, that's true."

"So what holds them here? Take this man O'Shaughnessy, for example. He's the middle one of three generations of O'Shaughnessys on the Mayo Clinic staff and he's damned near sixty years old—"

"Oh, you mean Ian?"

"Right," I said. "The little neurosurgeon. He's a fascinating guy. You know where I met him? I met him at the airport. I'd driven out there this afternoon late to check on the airlines that cover Rochester and get some idea of the flight schedules, and I'd heard there was a good place to eat there, and when I walked through the lobby I ran into this chap I *knew* I'd seen around the Clinic, so I stopped him and introduced myself. It was Dr. O'Shaughnessy. He and his wife had been out to the country club for an hour of golf when he'd finished his rounds and they'd stopped at the airport because it was the handiest place to stop for a drink on their way home to dinner." I looked up at Art. "Well, this man was a very sharp cookie," I said. "His daddy was a surgeon here before him and his son is coming up behind him in training here, and I would have quizzed him a lot more except that he was all keyed up about some crazy case that came in this afternoon and wasn't paying much attention. But I kept asking myself what it could be that keeps a guy like that at Mayo Clinic all these years? Do they really make all that much money?"

"Money? Not really. Their salaries are adequate but not terribly generous. I mean, they have enough to live on, enough to buy some decent clothes, enough to keep their wives happy and send their children to decent colleges—but they're not getting rich, if that's what you mean. The Mayo brothers set a standard, way back, and it still prevails: members of the Clinic staff should have a decent remuneration, an adequate remuneration, but any money generated beyond that would go into teaching and research. That's the way they started it and that's the way it's been ever since."

"So what does that mean in dollars and cents?" I said.

"I'm not going to quote salaries, if that's what you mean. The dollar amount doesn't mean much anyway, with the inflation that's going on. But I will say there probably isn't a man on the Clinic staff who couldn't earn three times as much somewhere else—on a big-city hospital staff or in private practice. But then what has he got? If he's in private practice he has to fight for patients, right? If he wants to bring in a really big income he's got to go to all the right functions, meet all the right people, please all the right VIPs. Well, we don't have to fight for patients here—our appointments are one or two steps ahead of us, most times. Then you take the guy with the big hospital and academic appointment. He'll get more money than a Mayo man, *lots* more money—but he's buried from the very start in a big, fat administrative hassle. He spends half his life writing applications for federal grants to get money to keep his department together—and his big salary coming in—for another year, and it's always only for another year. He can be deep in the middle of vastly important research and get cut off at the knees one day because the U.S. government in its infinite wisdom decides it isn't important any more and cuts off his grant money. Well, the man at Mayo here has all the research facilities he could ever ask for, and the money isn't likely to be cut off at a moment's notice. He may have to worry about applying for grants, too, since fifty-five percent of our research money comes from federal grants—but there's an awful lot of Mayo Clinic money to back him up in a pinch. All he's got to do is convince his colleagues that his work is worth the money he's spending—and that can be a whole lot easier than trying to convince Joe Califano."

Art leaned back in his chair and stared out the window at the tree-lined streets below. In many ways the town looked like a desert oasis: green and verdant, with the tree cover so thick that only here and there could you see a flicker of traffic or a group of people walking by on the street. "If you're trying to figure out what makes Mayo doctors tick, you can't just look at salary," he said finally. "I know you hear a lot of blather these days, most of it from power-hungry government officials and Senators, about how rich and fat and greedy all the doctors are, especially private doctors—but believe it or not, there are other things that matter more to most of them. The staff doctors here at Mayo have a maximum amount of freedom to do whatever they want to do in their special fields of medicine with very little of the stultifying paperwork and administrative hassle that most doctors these days have to put up with. In addition, our doctors enjoy some very significant fringe benefits. Naturally the health and medical needs of themselves and their families are covered at no cost to them. There are some very generous retirement provisions for the men who have worked here for years. As I said, they don't have to go looking for patients, but they aren't tied down to patients, either. As a matter of principle, the doctors work interchangeably. Part of the time a doctor will spend seeing patients in the Clinic. Then for a while he'll be relieved of Clinic duties in order to take care of patients in the hospitals, all on a regular rotation basis. Our doctors don't have to sit up all night three nights in a row because one patient is seriously ill—unless they want to. A doctor may well have quite a number of patients he's particularly interested in and wants to follow personally, but that's *his* choice, on *his* time. The minute he walks out the door to go home, somebody every bit as capable and competent and expert is on hand to take over.

"Among other things, this means he can enjoy real vacation time, thirty days a year. He can take it in pieces or all at one whack. All he needs to do is get his name on the chart so that too many people aren't gone from one department at one time. What's more, he can *take* that vacation without worrying about his practice going to hell while he's gone, the way other docs do. He can go when he feels he needs to the most. And figure this: If he's starving for theater or opera or ballet, New York is two hours away by air. Chicago is a half hour or so. Minneapolis is two hours' drive. St. Louis is just down the river a ways, and New Orleans isn't so much farther. They can even get to California or Hawaii without too much hassle if they're crazy enough to want to." Art grinned. "Of course most of them don't," he said. "Most of them go up to a cabin on some little lake up north to read and relax and do a little fishing. Some send their families up there for the whole summer—it gets pretty hot down here— and just fly up on weekends."

"What about medical meetings and things like that?" I asked.

"That's in addition to vacation time. Each staff man is allowed another eighteen days a year to attend medical conferences, all expenses paid. The doctors at Mayo are experts in their fields, and one of the ways they stay experts is by frequent contact with others who are also experts. Conferences let them keep up with whatever is brand new in their fields, and it gives them a chance to report their own research findings. Our people are constantly being invited to contribute to medical seminars, be guest speakers at medical meetings, go out to Boise, Idaho, and explain to the doctors there just what in the hell we're doing back here. There's a lot of teaching and a lot of learning that goes on at those conferences.

"Then, finally, there's Rochester itself," Art said. "It's kind of a sleepy little place, sure, but who needs a lot of wild excitement at home when your work is already exciting enough? We *do* have certain cultural activities that doctors and their wives are active in, as well as others. We have a live-wire Civic Theater and a darned good one. We have our own symphony orchestra and our own art center, both going concerns. And then Rochester is a lovely little town in its own way. It's got pretty good shops and stores. The streets are kept clean and the garbage gets collected when it's supposed to. There are good schools for the kids—not the greatest, maybe, but good solid schools. We have a competent fire department and a clean police department; you don't have to worry about your daughter being raped and slaughtered on the way home from the movies some night. Maybe the place is quiet and stuffy and old-fashioned, but then maybe that's the way the doctors here like it."

"You make it sound," I said, "as if they can do almost anything they want to any time they want—or as little as they want, for that matter. But meanwhile, somebody must be keeping the store."

"Oh, the store gets kept all right," Art said. "These doctors put in long, hard days, five days a week, like clockwork, and they have call weekends as well. But there's more to 'keeping the store' than just seeing patients. The great thing is, they have enormous freedom to choose for themselves what they want to *do* with their working time. Take a guy who really loves clinical medicine. He wants to see patients and nothing else. Well, he can spend a hundred percent of his time doing just that, with every kind of diagnostic aid and consultant known to man right here to help him do it well. He's also got the support of research people dreaming up new and better diagnostic methods, medicines or programs of treatment to make his work more effective. Those guys are right in the next building; if he wants to talk to one, he can pick up the phone and chew the fat with him any time of the day."

"What about teaching?" I said. "You told me the other day that that was as important at Mayo as the clinical practice."

Art nodded. "It's a long-standing tradition here. If another guy, also expert in his field of medicine or surgery, really wants to teach, he can spend a quarter or more of his time doing just that. We have our own medical school here, as well as our own School of Health Related Sciences and our School of Physical Therapy. We also have six hundred and eighty graduate doctors-in-training, most of them busy learning specialties and needing desperately to be taught. For a born teacher the place is paradise, and the teaching activities here make this one of the greatest centers of medical learning in the world."

"So clinical practice—seeing patients—and teaching are two legs of the three-legged stool you keep talking about," I said. "What's the third? Research?"

"Right," Art said. "It covers the spectrum here all the way from basic science research to special patient-treatment protocols. Suppose you have another Mayo doctor who really wants to work in research more than anything else. He can spend one hundred percent of his time in research, if he wants to—and quite a number do. He'll probably be paid less than the internist or the surgeon, but he isn't expected to crank out results like sausages, either. Medical research can be as simple as a clinical trial of a new treatment program for *lupus erythematosis* over at St. Mary's, or as complex as building a new kind of computerized multiple-exposure scanning device for examining coronary arteries. I'll have to get you over to see that little toy. Our prototype machine is going to cost us over fifteen million dollars before we're through—but if the guys can ever get it to work, it's going to revolutionize the diagnosis of heart disease."

"Guys like that must be spending full time in research," I said.

"Those particular guys, yes. Most of that team aren't even physicians—they're physicists and bioengineers and computer experts. But the doctor-researcher has his place too. If he can make a plausible scientific argument for some study he wants to do, he'll get the lab space to work in and as much time as he needs for the work. Actually, it isn't always as one-way-or-the-other as I'm making it sound. Most of the doctors divide their time. Virtually all of the docs seeing patients in the Clinic also teach, if only because they have doctors-in-training working right alongside them most of the time. Some of the best teachers in the place also spend much of their time in the Clinic seeing patients because they want to do both. Most of the staff get involved in research of some sort or another to one degree or another, even if it's only acting as a clinical consultant on a research protocol, keeping the research guys in touch with how their research is going to be affecting patients. Or, if a clinician has a more complicated research project under his hat, he may take six months' leave from Clinic duties and concentrate full time on the research until he wraps it up. Then he comes back to the Clinic to see patients again. It can work any way the doctors want it to work, and it works well. The only thing that could kill it would be if we had a bunch of deadheads in here. Of course, we *do* have a few of them, but very few indeed. They generally find themselves invited to leave before too long."

"It all sounds great," I said. "For the doctor."

"Well, you asked what kept the doctors here. There's lots more here for a doctor than just a dumb little town to live in. There's a terrific intellectual ferment going on here constantly, very sharp people continually stimulating other very sharp people and being stimulated in return."

"But this 'intellectual ferment' is pretty largely about medicine," I said.

"Of course," Art said, looking startled. "That's what Mayo Clinic is all about." He laughed. "What would you expect? Look, any time or place you get two doctors together, they're going to talk about medicine. You know that. They're not going to talk about opera or the current political regime in Italy. Hell, they may not even know for sure who the President is this year. But medicine—that they know. Of course, the men and women here are not quite all that narrow, either. We have one chap here who composes piano sonatas in his spare time. It's all this modern, atonal, dissonant music—sounds like a kangaroo in a kettle factory. But he performs his stuff with the Minneapolis Symphony. We have painters, history scholars, writers—even politicians. Pretty good politicians, as a matter of fact. Every now and then we have to send somebody back to Washington to cut some wild-eyed Senator down to size."

"But how does the patient fare, with all of this doctor-freedom you're telling me about?" I asked. "It sounds as if he must see one face one time and another face another and never knows who he might see next, for sure. You make it sound like the doctors are sort of interchangeable parts in some kind of huge machine."

Art looked uncomfortable. "In a way, you're right," he said. "It's been that way from the very first, and it's gotten more so the bigger we've grown. There was a time when people came to Rochester to have Will or Charlie Mayo operate on them—and Will or Charlie operated on them. Then later, patients came to have Will or Charlie operate on them, but somebody else operated on them because Will or Charlie was booked up and only had time to look in and say hello. Then later still, patients came to Mayo Clinic to be operated on and didn't have any idea who was going to operate on them, and neither Will nor Charlie looked in because they were already buried under their own operating schedules. It's still that way today. Some say it's our one overwhelming weakness—that the patient coming to Mayo Clinic can't count on the continuing one-to-one doctor-to-patient relationship that he has with his family doctor back home. Others say this is our one overriding strength—that everybody here is so good at his job that it doesn't *matter* what doctor you see; you'll end up in the hands of someone enormously competent to take care of your illness no matter what it may be."

"But if a patient comes back here again and again, there must be *some* kind of continuity," I said. "You can't just make him start all over every time he walks in the door. Especially if he's got some long-term continuing illness."

"Oh, there's continuity all right. For one thing, most patients who return *do* have a doctor they regard as 'their' doctor. They may call him for an appointment, or tell the office they want to see *him*. If he's at a conference or on vacation and the matter isn't urgent, they may elect to wait till he's back—but one way or another, they'll see him. It may not be much more than a brief social visit if their problem is outside his field, but even if he bounces the patient to somebody else, he'll be checking on progress from time to time."

Art leaned back, clasping his hands behind his head. "Maybe even more important, there's the matter of the medical record. You've seen our patient charts?"

"You mean these funny little eight-by-ten-inch packets that come in the plastic folders?"

"Right," Art said. "Well, to many patients those little plastic folders are the great unresolved mystery of the Mayo Clinic. You should see their faces sometimes! You'd think they were seeing black magic. Here's this woman sitting in Dr. A's office up in East Fourteen, watching him leaf through this chart of hers and scribble a note on it. She knows it's the same chart she had when she was here two years ago because she recognizes a splotch of green ink somebody spilled on the top medical-history sheet. She doesn't know how Dr. A got the chart—she imagines that some little attendant went down somewhere the day before she arrived, picked it off a storage shelf some place and then brought it up to East Fourteen on the elevator. Which, of course, is the way most places do it.

"Well, Dr. A tells her he wants her to go down to see Dr. B on West Four and she'd better hurry to catch him before he goes to lunch. So ten minutes later she's down on West Four talking to Dr. B in his office—and there on his desk is that same chart with the green splotch on it. So Dr. B makes some notes on one of the pages of the chart and then tells her that he wants her to go right over to the Medical Sciences Building and up to Dr. C's laboratory. She hustles along as fast as she can, but when she gets there, there's that chart with the green splotch sitting on Dr. C's desk. Now this could go on all day, and sometimes it does. Every place she goes, her chart seems to get there before she does. But *how?* There just *can't*

be some little attendant with that chart under her arm gal-
loping from floor to floor and building to building. So how
does it *get* there?"

"On fairies' wings?" I asked.

Art grinned his cadaverous grin. "Damn near it," he said.
"Maybe you don't remember the old-time department stores
back in the Twenties and Thirties, with only one person they
trusted with the money, up on the top floor somewhere, so
when the clerks at the counters collected money, they'd ship
the cash up to the cashier by vacuum tube. They'd just put
the money in a little brass capsule, shove the capsule into the
tube, yank the cord and away it went. And if there was
change due, a minute later, *wham!* there was the capsule
back again with the change in it. Well, we use the same
system for those funny little charts. They're designed to roll
up and fit into a large-size vacuum-tube capsule. A routing
slip goes in with the chart saying where it's supposed to go
next. It then gets lifted up to the top floor of the Mayo Building. If the routing slip says it's supposed to go to West Four,
the operator up there drops it down the chute for West Four
and *wham!* it's there. If it's supposed to go to the Medical
Sciences Building on a certain floor, she drops it down another chute, and *wham!* it's there. This whole place is hon-
eycombed with vacuum tubes—all of the Mayo complex and
Methodist Hospital and St. Mary's Hospital as well. The
chart bound for St. Mary's goes through an underground
tube one mile long in forty-five seconds flat. It's really incredible, because with this system the charts can move far faster
than the patient ever can. By the time a patient gets in to see
a doctor, the doctor not only has the chart on his desk but
he's had a chance to look at it already. He's also had time to
be on the phone to the doctor referring the patient, if he has
some question about what he's supposed to do."

"So essentially, every patient is squeezed down into an
eight-by-ten-inch chart," I said thoughtfully, "identified by a
seven-digit number."

"Well—everything that's medically important about the
patient is squeezed down into the chart, yes," Art said, giving
me an odd look, as if that were not precisely the image he had

meant to convey. "I mean, everything any doctor in the place needs to know about the patient up to the present moment is right there on those colored pages in the chart. And anything new he learns goes in there too. And it works."

It was certainly obvious that *something* worked. Yet clever and facile and eminently practical as Art Amundson made it all sound, I found myself uneasy as I rode the elevator back down to the lobby. I had this disquieting picture of a patient—a gray, faceless, anonymous, complex patient—disembodied like ectoplasm and compressed onto sheets of colored paper neatly encased in a plastic folder to be rolled into a cylinder and whisked away from here to Guinea in a vacuum tube. Whisk! No patient! He's gone to West 14—or all that matters about him has. I remembered accounts of African natives who were terrified of cameras because they thought their souls were stolen when their pictures were taken. And here at Mayo Clinic, were the patients' souls stolen and whisked off to West 14 in those plastic folders? A foolish question—but where was the *human* element in all this?

Morning hospital rounds on Dr. Howard Norgaard's service at St. Mary's Hospital were brisk affairs on his "orange days"—the alternate days each week when he was not scheduled for surgery in the operating room. These were the days that he spent primarily in the Clinic seeing patients in consultation, examining patients he would be operating on later, making diagnostic decisions or helping other doctors make them, seeing postoperative patients returning for follow-up, attending to a never-ending pile of correspondence, mostly to referring physicians outside the Clinic, which his secretary couldn't handle, or working on a paper he was scheduled to present at a heart surgeons' meeting three months hence. The paper dealt with a new technique he had devised for closing the inner lining of the heart to leave behind a smoother, less abrasive surface, thus reducing the chances of blood clots forming or bacterial infection taking root. He had used the technique now on more than forty successive open-heart patients and had sufficient postoperative follow-up to convince him that his new method led to significantly fewer grave complications than the older techniques that most heart surgeons were still using.

These Clinic days started at 7:30 in the morning, and Dr. Norgaard did not usually waste much time with his hospital rounds. He was at St. Mary's Hospital at twenty minutes of seven to meet Buzz Turnbull and four other Fellows, together with the new surgical intern (he still thought of them as "interns" even though now they were called "G-1s" or first-year graduate doctors), and found them all prepared for a brisk walk.

This particular morning he raced along more swiftly than usual—a brief check of a chart, a query about one patient's intake and output, another patient's respiration, the results of a urine check for pus cells, some bloody sputum, and so on. Buzz would be checking everything more thoroughly later and flag him if there were any headaches. He would smile and say hello to a patient, ask how he was feeling, scribble a brief note in the chart while the patient responded, and then whisk off to the next one. One doctor-in-training would stay behind to file the charts, while another rushed ahead to grab the next ones, and Dr. Norgaard moved along like a tall, wiry dynamo.

He realized suddenly that he was putting Manuela off for last, perhaps from a half-conscious desire to postpone the inevitable as long as possible, a certain feeling of dread that shadowed his mind whenever he thought about her. He had seen her the previous evening, after the surgery, and she'd looked awful then; but then they always looked awful the evening after surgery, and Charlie Hornby's crew was busy riding her hard. *He would have called me if she'd gone out during the night,* he thought. *He promised he'd call me if that happened. But then, it could have gotten lost. Things do get lost around this place.*

He found Hornby at the nurses' station in the intensive-care unit, bending over a desk and scribbling on a chart. "So how's our girl this morning?" Norgaard asked.

Hornby looked up gloomily. "She's still breathing," he said.

It didn't sound good. Charlie was usually far more enthusiastic when things were going well at this point. "At least that's something," he said. "But what's the trouble?"

Hornby sighed. "It was a dark and stormy night," he said. "Arrhythmias, man. You name it, she had it. Her heart has been going all over the place. Finally, about three o'clock this morning, she coughed up a plug of bronchial mucus as big as your thumb and turned a little pinker then, but before that she was gray as a foggy morning, only getting air to half a lung. And her blood pressure still wants to lie there like a dead dog. We just have to keep supporting it all the time." He shrugged. "I don't know, Howie, she just doesn't seem to have anything to work with. It's like trying to treat a wet dishrag. Nothing responds to anything."

"She's a very small, frightened, sick little girl," the surgeon said, "and she's just about literally been beaten to death—by surgeons. You can't expect her to snap back like Billie Jean King."

"No, but I sure hope she starts turning a corner somewhere along the line here, because I don't think we can prop her up much longer." Hornby glanced up at the row of TV monitors as he spoke. "Damn it, that heart rate is slipping out of control again. You want to see her? Come take a look."

As they walked into Manuela's room one of Hornby's Fellows was already adjusting an IV drip, and the arrhythmic heart rate, visible on the wall monitor, was once again settling down. Glancing at the girl herself, Norgaard would have been utterly appalled if he hadn't known what to expect. The child looked as if she'd been hit by a truck. Her color was a paste gray, with huge blue circles under the eyes. Tubes emerged from virtually every orifice in her body, and IV drips were going into both arms, mottled black and blue from elbow to wrist because of the difficulty the doctors had had finding veins at all. "Any fever?" the surgeon asked.

"Just a degree or so, thank God."

"What about neurological?"

"That's fine. She's perfectly alert and taking everything in—and I mean *everything*. There's no neurological loss at all that I can see, and she can respond. Ed Ruiz is in here babbling Spanish to her every free minute he can find. She seems to like that."

"See if you can't get him free for a day or two so he can be in here more," Norgaard said. *"I* like that too."

He walked over to the girl's bed and placed his stethoscope on the chest where the bandages allowed, then up at the base of the neck. Manuela turned her head away and stared at the wall. "Hey," he said softly, "Manuela." She didn't move. "Manuela! You know who I am?"

She looked at him accusingly and nodded once.

"I'm the guy who fixed up your heart."

She looked away at the wall again.

"How are you feeling?"

"Malo."

"Muy malo?"

"Muy, muy, muy malo," the girl said miserably.

"You aren't mad at me, are you?" Manuela just gave him a dirty look. "Well, *are* you?"

Something flared in the girl's dark eyes—scorn, indignation, contempt, loathing. "I hate you," she said with a flash of vigor.

"Why do you hate me?"

"You made me hurt."

Something touched the surgeon's mind and suddenly—suddenly—something clicked. "That's right," he said to her. "I *did* make you hurt. And it makes you mad to hurt. Well, that's all right. You go right ahead and hate me. I deserve it. Get real mad at me and real mad at hurting, too. Because if you get mad enough the hurting is going to get better."

He left the room then with the barest hint of a wink at Charlie Hornby and went on with his crew to see the last remaining patients. There were some others with problems, and there was a long hard day ahead, but it didn't matter now, because Howard Norgaard's day was already made. Charlie Hornby was crazy. That wasn't any wet dishrag lying there in that bed with all the tubes and monitors and busy doctors doing important things on all sides of her. That was one very tough little girl lying there, literally sick to death, but a whole lot tougher than she was sick, with one whale of a lot to work with, if they could just get her mad enough to fight. And if somehow she could just fight her way through the next twenty-four hours, she could have it made.

Q: What about uniform requirements at the Mayo Clinic? I don't mean the hospital nurses—that's pretty standard— but what about the Clinic personnel? The girls don't seem to be wearing uniforms exactly, yet they all seem to look alike.

A: We don't have any specific uniform, as such, except for the helpers in the lobby. They wear blue. But the Clinic aides do have some very distinct guidelines about dress—call it a dress code.

Q: I gather they can wear any color they want as long as it's white.

A: Yes, white is the favored color around here. But there are other things. It's made clear how long the skirts should be, how much bosom should be allowed to show, how much jewelry can be worn and of what kind, what kind of hose are acceptable. A girl may choose to break these rules—but after a bit she'll be invited to have a friendly discussion with her supervisor. If she still breaks the rules too flagrantly, she'll presently learn that the Clinic has had to cut back on its staff, and she is the one who's being cut back. It's as simple as that.

Q: Okay—but what about the doctors?

A: Again, there aren't any specific rules, just general attitudes. Considerations of what's appropriate and what isn't. The staff doctors wear business suits or fairly conservative sport coats and slacks—we don't go for the long white lab coat scene. The doctors also wear neckties, and they don't loosen them when the weather gets warm, either. We have pretty good air conditioning in here. Why neckties? Because the doctors think it's appropriate. The only ones who sometimes don't wear neckties are the surgeons going to the hospital for morning surgery—they're going to change into scrub suits first thing anyway. But they carry neckties in their jacket pockets, because they're going to make rounds on patients after the surgery is over. Oh yes, the doctors also wear shirts. And shoes. *Everyone* wears shoes at the Mayo Clinic. We consider it . . . appropriate.

The human element at the Mayo Clinic was the big hole in the picture, the part I could not quite pin down, yet I felt certain that it had to be there somewhere. No group of faceless, anonymous, interchangeable doctors, however expert they might be in their special fields, could substitute for the plain human contact of patient with doctor that I had always been taught was vital to any truly good medical care. Fancy laboratory facilities and nice, shiny diagnostic equipment were no substitute either, no matter how much they might tell about the functioning of the patient's physical body. The human element *had* to exist here somewhere. It *must* have been here when the Mayo brothers were alive—brilliant surgery alone could never have built this place—and it had to be here still, I was convinced, or the Mayo Clinic would long since have fallen down into ashes. Yet the human element continued to be the most elusive quarry of all in the course of my several visits to Rochester.

It had to be there—but where? I never did find it in a single chunk, just in bits and pieces here and there. One part of it showed up in the case of Millie Hulbert.

When Dr. Jerry Whitehead finished with his surgery on Millie, before even changing back to street clothes, he found a house phone and punched out a four-digit number to summon Tim MacMichael to the line. "Tim? Jerry here. I just finished doing Millie Hulbert and I thought you'd want a report."

"Yes, indeed," the older man said. "I've been waiting to hear."

"Well, I'm afraid it's a mixed bag," the surgeon said. "First the good news: The lump in her breast was *not* a recurrence of that melanoma she had on her leg sometime back. Pathology was sure of that from the frozen section."

"Thank God for that," Tim MacMichael said.

"Well, I was really worried on that score," Whitehead said. "You know how treacherous those damned things are, and if I'd found recurrent melanoma in her breast the fat would really have been in the fire."

"I know," MacMichael said dryly. "So now cheer me up some more and tell me it was just a benign cyst."

"I wish I could," the surgeon said, "but I can't. It was a primary breast carcinoma. Still very small, maybe one and a half centimeters, with no evidence of local invasion beyond that. In fact, it almost seemed encapsulated. Well, I certainly didn't want to do a radical mastectomy on a woman that age with that small a primary tumor, so what I did was essentially a wedge resection of the right upper quadrant. Closed the skin just fine. She won't have any significant deformity. And of course I had to go up into the axilla and snake out some of the nodes from there to see where we stood on distant spread."

"Yes, the nodes," MacMichael said. "What did you find?"

"I got seven nodes," Jerry Whitehead said. "Two of them had cancer in them."

"Oh dear," Tim MacMichael said. He was silent for a long moment. "I was afraid of that. So what do we do now, Jerry?"

"Tim, I really need your opinion in order to say," the surgeon replied. "You know the woman well; you've known her for years. If she were my mother, I know what I'd do. But she's not my mother."

"What would you do if she were your mother?"

"Nothing whatever until something showed up in her liver or lung or bone—and then play it by ear, as much or as little treatment as she can tolerate, but very gently."

"Tell me why you'd do that," the older man said.

The surgeon sighed. "Well, in the first place, I see here an eighty-year-old woman with a full life behind her, with excellent good health throughout most of it, widowed for years but with five grown children spread out all over the country, eleven grandchildren, some of them in college already. Not exactly a coherent family, but they care, and she has old, lifelong friends who also care. And even though her health has been good until recently, these next few years are the ones when a lot of different things can start falling apart fast. I spent quite a bit of time talking to her last evening, Tim. She's a strong-willed, opinionated woman. She doesn't care much for doctors, generally speaking, and she hates to take medicine and she doesn't like to feel sick one damned bit, and I sure would hate to start playing God with a woman like this."

"Go on," MacMichael said.

"All right, there's a long outside chance that I may already have gotten this cancer—all of it. It's not much of a chance. It's like walking in one night and breaking the bank at Caesar's Palace, but there's no reason she can't be encouraged to think the chances are better than that so she doesn't sit and stew about it—at least until her body starts telling her otherwise. Number two, there's also a reasonable chance that her body may contain and control whatever cancer remains, without any help, maybe for years, before it finally breaks loose and gets her. She could well have five or more comfortable, fruitful years before the bad time comes. She could *very* well die of something else in the meantime. Of course, maybe it won't go that way. Maybe it'll only be six months—but at least it could be a good comfortable six months."

Jerry paused. "Now, we did order an estrogen receptor assay from pathology on the tumor itself. We won't have an answer on that for a while—but if the cancer is estrogen-sensitive, we have an excellent chance for long-term palliation with these new antiestrogen drugs, when the time comes, and they're very nontoxic; they won't make her sick as a dog. On the other hand, if I were to send her down to the X-ray boys right now, or start feeding her cell poisons, or go flirting with the idea of an ovariectomy or adrenalectomy, there's no guarantee that any of these things are going to help her a bit, or add more than a few months to her survival, but there's an absolute guarantee that they're going to make her deathly ill and miserable and incapacitated for weeks or months at a time just from the treatment. Now, maybe you know some eighty-year-old woman who ought to have those things done to her, Tim, but somehow I don't think *this* woman should. I think she's going to do better without it. Maybe not much better, but not much worse either."

There was a long silence over the telephone, and then Tim MacMichael took a deep breath. "Well, Jerry," he said, "you have my blessing. I think Millie might take it and keep on taking it a whole lot better than you think. But she'd hate every minute of it, and very soon she'd be wishing desperately that she *wasn't* taking it, that she'd just told us to go hang. And what kind of quality of life would *that* be? I say be conservative and be gentle. Just follow her closely enough that you know when she needs help." The older man paused. "Of course, when push comes to shove, *she's* the one who's got to do the deciding. Do you want me to talk to her?"

"She's certainly going to want to see you," Jerry Whitehead said. "She'll be out of recovery and back in her room by this evening. But I already talked to her at some length last night before the surgery. Just sort of laid out the options, what we might find, what we'd probably recommend if we found this or that, what this or that finding might mean and which direction to go from there. Her attitude then was pretty much for me to try to kill the damned thing if I could, but if I couldn't, then to do as little beyond the surgery as made sense. If you approve, I'll see her this evening myself and explain what we found, tell her what the options are and see what she wants to do."

"Well, I approve," the older man said, "but I already know which way she's going to go. I'll see you later, Jerry."

As the surgeon went back to change into his street clothes for rounds, Tim MacMichael sat back in his chair, feeling a vast wave of depression. *It would have to be that way, wouldn't it?* he thought. *Miserable, hateful disease. But people don't go on forever, and the doctor's job is to help, not to force.* Sitting there, he had a sudden fleeting image of times long past and forgotten, of Millie Hulbert as a young woman with her husband up at the lake in the summer, the kids swarming all over the beach, struggling with a rowboat, pulling up sunfish by the dozen or exuberant at finding a crappie hole. A woman who later was stricken but still strong at her husband's sudden and untimely death—just forty-three, George was, when he went—and Millie digging in and raising those kids but letting them go gracefully when the time came. The older doctor shook his head and sat up, glancing at his call board that showed him where his next patient was, and he suddenly found the sense of depression was gone. *You old fool,* he thought to himself, *what are you fretting about? Millie Hulbert is going to see you in your grave, and you damned well know it, too.*

The human element. I did not quite find it in the course of my own complete physical examination at the Mayo Clinic, although I found other things. I found competence, immense skill, meticulous thoroughness and more than a little medical wisdom brought to bear during that examination. Even more welcome, I found some answers to medical problems I had been looking for for years—but not the elusive human touch I thought I might find.

From the first it had seemed slightly ridiculous to try to write about patients at the Mayo Clinic without actually being a patient there myself—so early on I "signed myself into the Clinic," as the saying goes. There was nothing covert about it—the Clinic knew who I was and what I was doing there—but there was nothing red-carpet about it, either. They were overcrowded at that particular time, and since they could see that I was not actively hemorrhaging, they set up a formal appointment to coincide with my next planned visit to Rochester two months later. It was then that my personal adventure in the great gray building began—no sooner and no later.

Of course, my appointment was not entirely a matter of snooping. Though I was in reasonably good health, I did have certain real medical problems that needed dealing with. I weighed too much, enjoyed all the wrong foods and still smoked cigarettes. My blood pressure was a trifle too high in spite of simple medication I was taking to control it. Most irritating of all, I had also had periodic episodes of depression over the years that lasted far too long when they came and failed to respond very well to my regular doctor's ministrations.

The Mayo doctors dug in, as they would with any patient. I was first assigned to see Dr. Dan Fogarty, a cardiologist—possibly, I thought, because I looked like a prime candidate for a coronary at any minute. Fogarty was an elderly, gentlemanly sort who looked so very much the perfect image of a

Mayo Clinic physician that he might have been stuffed and sent to the Smithsonian. He was painstakingly thorough in reviewing my medical history—so smoothly, unerringly thorough that I hardly realized at the time what an incredibly *slick* job he was doing. No one but a doctor can appreciate the truly vital importance of a medical history in getting to the bottom of a patient's health problems, and nobody but a doctor can appreciate the sheer artistry that goes into eliciting a *thorough* history. When the patient is also a doctor, the ground is even more treacherous; doctors and their families are the most prone of all to turn up with bizarre, unthinkable or disastrous diagnoses, as anyone in medicine well knows. Yet Dr. Fogarty faced this threat with no sign of discomfiture, calmly and placidly proceeding to leave no stone unturned.

Next, he conducted as exhaustive a physical examination as I have ever been subjected to before settling down to outline the studies he felt to be indicated in the next stage of the diagnostic process—the part most patients are referring to when they speak of "going through the Clinic." All in all, that history and physical exam was a virtuoso performance in every way, yet strange to say, I ended up feeling quite certain that a baboon presenting itself at the Clinic appointment desk and assigned to Dr. Fogarty would have been afforded precisely the same meticulous examination that I had received. The human element, the sense of contact with another concerned human being, was not quite there. Almost but not quite.

Various studies and consultations occupied the following three days, off and on. Like every other Mayo patient, I paid my personal visit to the infamous Desk C. I received my plastic jugs and jars to carry around with me in their paper bags, in regard to which I was cheerfully given instructions I shall forbear to repeat. I had been found to have a small blistery affair on the sole of one foot, so I encountered a dermatologist who examined it, studied it, scraped it, cultured it and viewed stained smears of it before prescribing an ointment for it, although something told me it was just a little athlete's foot.

Later, like Roger Barton, I too had a meeting with the charming blonde in the Blood Pressure Laboratory, got hooked up to the automatic pressure measurement machine and spent half an hour watching the second hand creep slowly around the clock. Still later I discussed my blood pressure with Dr. Weakner, a small, brisk man of forty-five with half-glasses and a sly little smile that kept creeping up to his eyes as he outlined some minor modifications of medicine that might help keep my pressure better subdued without turning me into a zombie. We got along fine as long as the conversation remained in precisely the channels he chose—but it was soon evident that those channels were very narrow. He was not interested in discussing the general problems of blood-pressure medications, nor any possible awkward side effects that I was not actively suffering at the moment, nor anything else of the sort. Only once did Dr. Weakner lose his composure for moment. He was warning me that one medicine he was considering for me often caused people to have bizarre dreams. I told him that was fine; I enjoyed bizarre dreams. He stopped with his mouth open. "You *what?*"

"I *like* weird dreams," I said. "They make the nights more interesting. I sometimes even use them in stories."

For a long moment he just looked at me, as if I were about to bite him. Then he turned to my chart and abruptly got the conversation back onto less boggy ground. It was as if a complex computer had suddenly gotten into territory for which it wasn't programmed and consequently just *didn't know what to do*. I concluded that bizarre dreams were considered Bad in Rochester, Minnesota.

The psychiatrist I was scheduled to consult seemed similarly once-and-a-half removed from really direct contact with his patient. Like everyone else I saw, he was thorough almost to a fault. He did not seem bound to the classical fifty-minute hour which reigns throughout the rest of the world of psychiatry. He took a detailed history of the depressive episodes I had been having, starting (I guess logically enough) at my birth and working forward from there. When we reached the point of recent and current problems his rapid note-taking accelerated and he began asking specific questions: drinking habits, other drugs licit or illicit, disturbances in sleep, disturbances in sex function, disturbances in work habits, problems with antidepressant medications previously prescribed, any *patterns* of depression I had noticed and whether they had recurred and if so in what way. Finally, with infuriating exuberance and good cheer, he said, "Well, my goodness! This is very, *very* interesting! Absolutely fascinating!"

"*I* don't think it's so fascinating," I said. "*I* think it's a pain in the ass."

He looked startled. "Well—from *your* point of view, I suppose it is. But as a clinical problem, it presents some extremely interesting points. You see, you've been treated right along as if this were an ordinary exogenous depression—that is, as if you were depressed because of outside influences pressing in on you until you couldn't cope. I dare say you've been assuming that yourself. But the things you're telling me here aren't really consistent with that kind of depression at all. One really would have to think about an endogenous depression—an internal, chemical sort of thing that has nothing to do with external problems. And that might suggest a totally different approach to treatment which might perhaps give far more satisfactory results—"

And so it went. Later, in a final wrap-up interview with Dr. Fogarty, the many pieces of my four-day examination were fitted together in neat order, reviewed and assessed. Only then were specific recommendations made. Medication was ordered which I could tolerate but which would also control my borderline high blood pressure as simply as possible. A psychiatrist in my own city was recommended to monitor the new treatment approach to my depression (an approach which literally hit the nail on the head; I only wish someone had thought of it ten years ago). Dr. Fogarty indicated that further follow-up with Mayo doctors was unnecessary unless I wanted it but that he stood ready to help at any future time if I so desired. He shook my hand with a pleasant goodbye, and I went on my way after picking up my formal discharge and my own personal Mayo Clinic Identification

Card certifying in sturdy plastic that I and I alone was the Clinic's 3,266,241st patient, a number no other human will ever share with me.

And through it all, from beginning to end, I had been aware of a curious sense of detachment in the Mayo doctors and personnel, as if a closely coordinated set of educated, even brilliant, eyes had been busily examining a sometimes interesting specimen under a glass, finding it wanting in certain areas, making the necessary repairs, recording what had been discovered and what had been done and then moving it along to make way for the next possibly interesting specimen. The human element? Here and there I almost sensed it, but never quite. Yet human element or no, *these people had found answers that other fine physicians had not found.* Which did I prefer—a totally comfortable, reassuring human element, or answers to some very distressing problems? If one had to take his choice, I think there are times when one might much rather have the answers.

About the time that Millie Hulbert was being wheeled out of the surgical recovery room and up to her semiprivate room on the fourth floor of Rochester Methodist Hospital, Roger Barton turned up at the laboratory office of Dr. Gerald Fried in the Medical Sciences Building. He'd been offered the choice of seeing Dr. Fried in his office or having Dr. Fried come over to the Clinic to see him at Dr. DeVore's office, but he had elected the former. *Since I'm here, I might as well see what all this famous Mayo research money is being spent for,* Roger thought. *See what these weird chaps do over here with their beakers and test tubes and all.*

Unfortunately, the "laboratory" of Dr. Fried was a bit of a disappointment. It consisted of a grubby little hole-in-the-wall office, so dingy and lightless, with its one small window in this ancient building, that the overhead lights had to be on at high noon on a bright, sunny day. Wall shelves and floors were stacked high with piles of books, journals and papers, some with quite visible dust on them. There was an old upholstered swivel chair with the stuffing coming out of it for the doctor to sit on and a huge old-fashioned rolltop desk (*damn thing must be worth a small fortune*, Roger reflected) with every possible nook and cranny of it stuffed with papers and scribbled-on sheets from a yellow legal tablet. There were no signs of any test tubes or beakers. Dr. Fried was certainly a weird-looking little chap, only five feet tall, skinny as a shadow in profile, with a large head, a deep widow's peak and an enormous nose he seemed to scratch constantly. "Glad to see you," he told Roger, scooping a couple of books off the hard straight chair beside his desk and offering it as a seat. (The books went onto the floor in another corner of the room.) "I've been talking to Earl De-Vore about your situation several times and I've been anxious to meet you." He leafed through the now familiar chart in the plastic folder sitting on his desk. (*My albatross*, Roger thought gloomily. *I can't get rid of it.*) "Yes, I've been *very* eager to talk to you. You know, you're quite an unusual young man."

This was hardly news to Roger Barton, but he settled himself smugly into the hard chair and smiled. "You mean because of my allergy to antihistamines?"

"Let's say, ah, because of your *reaction* to antihistamines," Dr. Fried said. "Or rather, your lack of it. You're certainly a highly allergic person. The tests show that without any doubt—as if we needed any tests, considering your history. You're one of these people with a nasal allergy to a whole lot of things and other things which trigger an asthmatic response—a sort of double-barreled effect in two organ systems, a vicious cycle for which we need precisely the right key in order to break the cycle. I think Dr. DeVore has some very interesting ideas about dealing with this kind of problem, and he's confident he can suggest some things to help you get it stopped, really break its back."

"I hope you're right," Roger said.

"Well, *I'm* rather excited, because I think what he's thinking might fit in with some studies I'm doing, if you'd be willing to take part."

"What kind of studies?" Roger asked suspiciously.

"Laboratory studies and medication studies," Dr. Fried said. He leaned back in his chair, staring up at the ceiling, which seemed to have a large cobweb from the overhead light to the wall. "You speak about being 'allergic' to antihistamines, but I rather doubt that's really true." He shook his head to cut off Roger's protest. "I know that that's what it *seems* like," he said. "You start having symptoms of your nasal allergy, so you pop down a couple of antihistamines and the symptoms get worse instead of better, and you say to yourself, 'Aha, I'm allergic to antihistamines.' It makes perfect sense. Any intelligent person might figure it that way. And it's possible—barely. But what's far more likely is that you're simply *fast* to antihistamines."

"Fast?" Roger said.

"Unresponsive. Deadhead. You take them and they have no effect whatever any more. After all, you've been eating them like popcorn since you were a kid. What happens is that you begin a cycle of symptoms and take the antihistamines and they have no effect whatever and the cycle of symptoms goes right on as if you hadn't taken anything at all. Then pretty soon you're not only in the soup with your nose, you're in the soup with your chest too. Okay, we believe that people who have this response have something different going on in their bodies' immune systems than people who don't. We think one measure of this difference is the presence of certain special kinds of white blood cells known as eosinophils leaking out of the bloodstream into allergic areas such as the nose and the lungs. We think by measuring changes in the numbers of these cells from specimens of mucus we take from those two areas we can perhaps detect individuals with your particular kind of trouble very early and maybe get started with special treatments very early. So one part of what I have in mind is getting a series of nasal smears and sputum specimens from you over the next several months at regular intervals, both while you're having symptoms and while you're not. We can get the first samples while you're here and get later ones when you return here for follow-up—or your doctor back home can collect the samples and mail them to us."

"My doctor back home can't grab his ass with both hands," Roger said. "I'd just as soon come back up here, if it isn't too often. But what is all this going to cost?"

"There'll be no cost to you," Dr. Fried said, "and maybe

no direct benefit, either. I just don't know that yet. But it can't do you any harm, and it *is* an opportunity for you to contribute a little bit to our knowledge about an exceedingly nasty kind of illness—as nobody knows better than yourself."

The little man hopped from his chair and searched through a pile of journals. "There's a paper here somewhere that would tell you more about it, but I can't seem to find it right now. Well, anyway, there's another part of my study that might benefit you more directly and would also cost you nothing. Dr. DeVore has in mind treating your condition with a new medicine we've found often helps allergic people, especially those who have become generally resistant to other drugs. I'm studying a sort of second generation of the same kind of medicine, so new that we're just now starting clinical trials with it on patients. I *think* this new drug may be two to three times more effective than the one Dr. DeVore is using and may only require about one fifth as much medicine, which would mean far less chance of side effects. Unfortunately, thinking isn't knowing. We need to actually *measure* the difference in human patients. We think it's remarkably well tolerated, too, but we don't know *that* for sure, either— and we need to find out. To do that, we've set up what we call a double-blind study with a large group of patients like yourself."

The doctor explained how it worked. Roger would be started on Dr. DeVore's medicine in any case, since he needed active, reliable treatment for his allergies and asthma right now. In addition, two other sets of pills would be prepared, looking exactly alike but a different color and shape from Dr. DeVore's medicine. One set would actually be the new medicine Dr. Fried was investigating. The other set would be placebos—sugar pills. Both kinds would be put in separate envelopes marked with code numbers by someone completely apart from the study, and the code would then be locked in the safe, so that neither the patient nor Dr. Fried would know which of the two kinds of pills any given patient was taking.

"Then we keep careful records of the responses all these patients have to their medicine, whatever it may be, throughout a full year, both during the high allergy season and in periods of low allergy trouble as well. We tell you what things we're looking for, what things we want *you* to mark down. At the end of the year's period we break the code and see what medicine did what for whom."

"Then I'd either be getting two allergy medicines, or just one plus a sugar pill," Roger said.

"That's right."

"But I wouldn't know which it was."

"No, you wouldn't. Neither would I—except possibly by the way your symptoms were behaving."

"And at least I'd be getting the stuff Dr. DeVore is planning to give me anyway."

"Right. Of course, you could drop out of the study any time you felt like it, but we'd rather you not start if you're considering that. You could also mess the study up something awful if you forget to take the pills off and on. We have to count on real cooperation from the patients, and we do supply the medicine without cost. What's more, you have a certain self-interest to consider. The study could well produce one of the most potent and effective antiallergic medicines that's ever been discovered—and we would certainly want patients in this study to have access to it at the earliest possible moment, if it proves as good as we think." Dr. Fried grinned broadly. "So you see, we have everything all figured out."

"So I see," Roger said sourly. "So when do you have to know?"

"Soon, but not this very instant," the researcher said. "I'd much rather you gave it some careful thought before deciding."

"Well, that I will do," Roger said, getting up from his chair. "Yes, I certainly will. I'll give it some very careful thought."

A beautiful early-summer afternoon in Rochester, Minnesota. Too many hours in a stuffy motel room working over my notes. I decided to take a walk out in the fresh air and sun, around the Clinic complex.

It was almost five in the afternoon. After three straight days of steaming heat and cloudless skies, with temperatures well over 100, thunderheads had piled up over the city about two o'clock in roiling black billows and let loose a glorious, crashing thunderstorm and downpour. Now the clouds were departing to the west, and sun was flooding the town with that special shimmering yellow-golden-green light so common to Midwest summer afternoons. The streets were glistening wet, water still rushing in the gutters, the air sweet and musty warm.

I walked down the street across from the Mayo Building, then stopped in the shade of the small and aged Heritage House Hotel on the corner to watch a crew of window washers hoisted up on a scaffold almost to the top of the Mayo Building. I'd seen them up there earlier in the day from my motel-room window, working away, and then lowering themselves hastily as the thunderstorm had built up. Now they were back up there again for a bit more work before quitting time.

I watched awhile and was starting to walk on when something peculiar struck me—something so *very* odd I was amazed I hadn't noticed it before. Those men up there *had* to be window washers—*but there weren't any windows on that side of the Mayo Building.* Nothing but the smooth, unbroken façade of neatly patterned gray granite blocks.

I watched, bemused, as the men worked away. They were up about the seventeenth-floor level, lowering themselves down a notch every now and then. In a little while they set aside whatever they were working with and began dropping the scaffold back down to the ground, their day's work obviously done. I walked across the street, determined to see what on *earth* they had on that scaffold with them. What they had were huge buckets of soapy water and huge buckets of clear water and long-handled, stiff-bristled brushes.

They were certainly window washers, but they were not washing windows. They were scrubbing down and polishing the outside of the Mayo Building.

The human element at the Mayo Clinic. It had to be somewhere, but I couldn't quite see where. It was certainly nowhere in evidence in the case of Sarah Swedman. *That* case was a total disaster for patient and Clinic doctors alike, precisely because of the *lack* of a human element.

She presented herself about 8:00 P.M. Thursday in the Emergency Room of Rochester Methodist Hospital, a thin, pale woman of about thirty-five. "I'm Sarah Swedman," she said to the young man on duty. "I'm supposed to be admitted for Dr. Sandleman."

"Dr. Sandleman?" The young doctor was a G-1 or intern, just beginning his first year of postgraduate medical training after medical school. He'd heard Dr. Sandleman's name somewhere, but there were a million names around this place. Dr. Sandleman. He ran his finger down a roster. "What department is he in?"

"The bowel department," the woman said. "I'm supposed to be admitted."

"Dr. Sandleman," the intern said. "Yeah, here's a Dr. Henry Sandleman."

"That's the one," Mrs. Swedman said. "The older Dr. Henry Sandleman, not the younger. He's been taking care of my bowel for years."

"Well, he's not on hospital service now," the young doctor said. "You'll have to go over to the Clinic."

"I just *was* over at the Clinic," the woman said. "The Clinic was closed, so they sent me over here. I'm supposed to be admitted for Dr. Sandleman."

The intern looked at her for the first time. She certainly looked sick enough. Everything about her looked washed out: her faded reddish hair, her broad, flat Scandinavian features, her pasty complexion, her very pale, watery blue eyes and a nose reddened at the end as though she was constantly sniffling. "When did you see Dr. Sandleman last— and what for?" the intern asked her.

"Oh, I've been seeing Dr. Sandleman for years. I've got this ulcerative colitis thing that goes on and on and he's been doctoring me. He even had the surgeons cut out a piece of my bowel a couple of times. But it didn't do no good. I keep having these attacks when I can't stop going, you know? With a lot of water and blood too. I knew a spell was comin' on, so I called him on the telephone last week, long distance from Faribault I called him, and he said if it got too bad, come on back to Rochester and he'd put me in the hospital again. Well, it's got too bad all right. I just about pass out every time I stand up, so I come in like he said." Her voice sounded whiny and self-pitying. "So here I am."

"Look, lady, I can't admit you to the hospital without authorization from the attending, and Dr. Sandleman isn't attending on the GI service right now. Dr. Millikan is attending."

"I don't want to see that Dr. Millikan," the woman said. "I've seen him before and he's no good. He thinks it's all in my head, though he won't say so straight out. It's Dr. Sandleman I want to see. Last week on the phone he told me to come right in and they'd put me to bed."

"But I just told you—"

"Look, Doctor, my husband just drove me all the way here from Faribault, and I'm about to fall on my face from the pain and all these stools and all, and I'm *telling you* what Dr. Sandleman said."

Defeated and a little bewildered, the intern sighed and pulled out some papers. "I suppose we can send you upstairs," he said, "and get Dr. Sandleman to see you in the morning. Meanwhile, one of the Fellows can see what you need right now." He started on the necessary paperwork, buzzed for the admitting nurse, ordered the woman's chart over.

"That's all right," the woman said. "I don't mind about a Fellow seeing me, as long as it's not Dr. Millikan and as long as I see Dr. Sandleman too. He told me to come right in. . . ." She was still talking in that same whiny voice, repeating the same phrases over and over as the admitting nurse whisked her down the corridor into an elevator for the sixth floor.

Sarah Swedman was certainly ill, and she certainly needed to be in the hospital. But she was *not* going to see Dr. Sandleman, because Dr. Sandleman was 5,000 miles away right then, touring ancient castles on the Rhine, and he was not going to be back in Rochester until his thirty-day vacation was over. What *did* happen to Sarah Swedman turned out to be one of the more spectacular messes in the recent annals of Mayo Clinic medicine.

The first thing that happened to Mrs. Swedman, stored away in her semiprivate room on the sixth floor of Rochester Memorial Hospital, which was costing her $86 a day plus extras, against which her husband's cut-rate "bargain" health insurance would pay only $27 a day, was that she was not seen at all by *anyone* with any significant degree of medical authority for three and a half days. True, a G-1 and a G-2 saw her the evening she was admitted, checked her voluminous chart in its little plastic folder and saw Dr. Sandleman's hastily scrawled note regarding last week's phone call: "To be admitted Methodist PRN care of attending." Between them the G-1 and the G-2 couldn't even be sure if she was on the right floor or not. "This is medical up here," one of them said. "But she was on surgical last time she was in. Dan Halar took out seven inches of her large bowel. Found some anaplasia or very early Ca in the specimen, too, it says here. Looks like she's got it bad."

"Yeah, but Sandleman didn't say which attending was supposed to see her."

"True. Well, she doesn't seem to be dying right now. Let's just put her in a holding pattern, slap her some routine orders and a sleeper and let Millikan decide what to do tomorrow morning."

That was Thursday night. Friday morning was just Dr. Millikan's second morning as attending on the gastrointestinal service; he had been hastily transferred from his Clinic duties when Dr. Sandleman had unexpectedly taken off for Europe. The GI service at that time happened to have a number of very sick patients demanding lots of attention, including a severe GI bleeder who wouldn't quit and upon whom the surgeons didn't want to operate until he was stabilized. Millikan was buried up to his ears in trouble by the time he'd been on the hospital floor ten minutes, trying to figure out who was doing what for whom, and he wasn't really getting his feet on the ground until noon. He had left his Chief Fellow, a sharp and experienced young chap, wrestling with the bleeder and had only a vastly inexperienced G-1 and a rather dull and unreliable G-2 to continue rounds with him. He had thought he was finished when the G-2 said, "Oh, yeah, there's one more" and handed him Sarah Swedman's chart.

"Who the hell is this?"

"Beats me," the G-2 said. "She just turned up during the night. She's a colitis patient Dr. Sandleman has been seeing."

"Oh, Christ," Dr. Millikan said. They were standing in a group well outside Sarah Swedman's door. "Crohn's disease, yet, as if I don't have enough grief already. Hmm. Swedman. I've seen this one somewhere. The name rings a bell. Is anything going on with her?"

"Not that I can see," the G-2 said. "She's having a flare-up, some diarrhea, and a little bloody stool. She says Dr. Sandleman told her to come in if she started having symptoms."

"Yeah, that's Sandleman for you," Millikan said. "Sending in one of *these* beauties and then grabbing the next plane to Europe." He sighed and poked through the chart. The last thing in the world he wanted just then was to tackle an ulcerative colitis patient with an acute flare-up. Then suddenly he stopped and read half a page. "Well, *hell*," he said. "She doesn't belong on this service anyway. She's a surgical problem. They've been whittling away on her bowel for the last five years! Find out who the surgical attending is and give him a call. Tell him we're transferring her to surgical. Meanwhile, just get her on a low-residue diet and find out what medicine Sandleman's been giving her, and let it go at that. Just order the barest routine. Then if the surgeons want to change things, they can change things. But let them be the first to see her. These people are like tar babies—once you touch them personally, you're stuck with them for the duration. Mike, you look in and say hello, will you? I'm already late for a committee meeting."

Dr. Millikan took off, and the G-2 stepped into Mrs. Swedman's room with a perfunctory greeting. Twice, as he stood scribbling notes in her chart, the woman asked in her whiny, piteous voice just when Dr. Sandleman was going to see her, but the G-2 just shook his head and went on writing. He was trying to figure out what "the barest routine" orders might be for ulcerative colitis patients, having never actually dealt with one before. *Probably better get her down for proctoscopy*, he thought, groping his way. *Find out what's going on in there. And a colon X ray too, I guess; probably can't do any harm.*

Finally he flashed Mrs. Swedman a smile and prepared for a swift exit. He did *not* mention that Dr. Sandleman was not going to see her at all, nor even one of his medical colleagues, nor did he mention that some surgeon was going to be seeing her instead. He didn't mention anything. He merely closed her chart with a snap and said, with splendid insincerity, "Okay, Mrs. Swedman, you just quit worrying. We're going to get you fixed up in no time" and hustled off about his business.

By this time Dr. James Towne, the surgical staff man in attendance on the hospital gastroenterology service, had already left the hospital after morning rounds. He was now over at the Clinic building catching up on correspondence before starting on his list of patients to see in consultation that afternoon. Mrs. Swedman's nurses dutifully set about following the G-2's orders, starting with the preparatory enema that was normally given before a proctoscopic examination. For this they hustled Mr. Swedman out of the room, ignoring his query about when Dr. Sandleman was going to be in to see his wife. Presently they trundled the patient down for her proctoscopy, an examination which literally terrified the woman because she knew from long experience that it would be excruciatingly painful. It was done without too much finesse by a bored G-3 who had already done seventeen of them that day and was mostly concerned with getting that fifteen-centimeter-long steel tube up Mrs. Swedman's rectum and back out again just as fast as he could. After she was taken back to her room, weeping silently, with violent abdominal cramps, they then transported her down for a colon X ray, only slightly more painful to her than the proctoscopy, even though it was performed with greater skill.

At evening hospital rounds Dr. Towne, the surgical staff

man, came to Mrs. Swedman's floor weary and unreceptive. He'd spent the afternoon at a dead run seeing consultation patients, overbooked as usual, with some thoroughly nasty surgical problems to sort out, and he very much wanted to get home, have dinner and spend the evening tinkering in his shop. Attended by his own crew of G-3s, G-2s and G-1s, he came to Mrs. Swedman last of all. But before stepping into her room, he stopped suddenly. "Say, tell me: Why am *I* seeing this patient?" he asked the Fellows. "She was on the medical service this morning."

"Beats me," said the G-2. "Dr. Millikan said transfer, so they transferred."

"Great," Dr. Towne said. "And I first hear about it at six-thirty on Friday evening. Well, let's see what it says here." He stood poring over Mrs. Swedman's chart for several long moments. "Well, hell," he said finally. "There's nothing going on with this woman that requires a surgeon at six-thirty on a Friday night. With all that diarrhea, we'd probably better check her electrolytes, get her on intake-and-output and get some Ringer's solution into her IV. And I suppose I'd better look in—"

He would have, too, except that at that moment his beeper sounded, and it was the Emergency Room. Some farmer had gone berserk and shot his wife with a deer rifle, and she was down there bleeding vigorously from several newly created orifices, and they needed Dr. Towne in surgery stat because they thought one slug might have grazed the abdominal vena cava or gone through her liver or something, and she was clearly going to need some fast attention. That fast attention took four solid hours in the operating room and left Dr. Towne wrung out and exhausted. When he finished there, he packed off for home, having completely forgotten about Mrs. Swedman on the sixth floor.

Over the weekend, of course, nobody did anything that didn't have to be done. The house doctors—all the G-1s, G-2s, G-3s and G-4s—were down to a bare maintenance crew to hold the fort against emergencies so the rest of them could have the weekend off for rest and recuperation. The Clinic doctors, for the most part, were off to their summer cabins or down to the river boating or out in the fields training their hunting dogs, leaving only those few with the bad luck to pull call that weekend hanging around Rochester waiting for the phone to ring. Neither Dr. Millikan nor Dr. Towne was on call. The Clinic itself, of course, was closed, and there was only a fragmentary Saturday-morning operating schedule in either of the hospitals.

Thus no one but a totally unfamiliar house doctor saw Mrs. Swedman on Saturday or Sunday, nor was anything in particular done about her condition, even though her basic bill at Rochester Methodist Hospital was still increasing inexorably to the tune of $86 a day. And as she grew more gloomy and morose by the hour and had more and more cramping and watery stools mixed with blood, her husband grew more and more restive, sitting in the room with her hour after hour.

It was about two o'clock on Monday morning, long after her husband had finally left for the boardinghouse room where he was staying, long after Dr. Steinman, the Clinic surgeon on call for the gastrointestinal service, had retired for a hopefully unbroken night of sleep, long after the interns and residents had departed to their individual nooks and crannies, hoping that another long duty weekend was finally wrapped up, and the night nurse on duty on Mrs. Swedman's unit was bracing herself for the long, dismal stretch between two and seven in the morning—it was then that Mrs. Sarah Swedman began bleeding from the bowel.

She did not mess around about it. She began bleeding a gusher. Normally a sad, inadequate, hopelessly incompetent woman, she was now doing an altogether too competent job of bleeding. Lying awake in her bed (she seldom slept more than an hour at a time anyway), she suddenly and involuntarily passed a lump of chalky paste from Friday's colon X ray and suddenly found herself lying in a pool of warm, wet, sticky stuff in the bed. She knew what it was; she'd been there before. Terrified, she called for the nurse, but could barely emit a croak from her dry throat. She groped frantically for the call button pinned to the mattress but couldn't find it; somehow it had slipped off the edge of the bed and was hanging down completely out of reach. She rolled out of bed, felt blood running down both legs, staggered to the door, felt her head spinning wildly, and then collapsed with a sickening thud, blood splattering all over, in front of a horrified nurse.

The nurse called the first doctor she could find, a G-2 she knew was still down on the fourth floor. Then she carried Sarah across to another room and got her into a clean bed while the G-2 was en route. He took one look from the door of the room and sent an aide to call Dr. Steinman, the surgical attending, while he and the nurse went to work fighting shock, getting the woman in Trendelenburg position with head low and feet high, getting another IV started in her vein, getting blood drawn for typing and crossmatch for transfusion and breathing a sigh of relief when the woman fluttered her eyelids and began to come around, still bleeding but at least responsive. Meanwhile, Dr. Steinman, jerked from his sleep at home, wasted no time getting across town to the hospital. He walked onto the floor, surveyed the carnage and said, "What in blazes is going on here?"

"I don't know," the G-2 said. "She's got colitis and she started bleeding, so they called me. I never even saw the woman before."

"It looks to me like nobody else has either," Dr. Steinman said. He looked closer at the chart and his jaw dropped. "Oh, wow," he said. "This woman came in here on Thursday night, and it's now Monday morning, and *nobody has even seen her*. She came in on Medicine, and Medicine gave her to Surgery without even looking at her, and Surgery—Surgery—what *about* Surgery? There's not even a *note* from Surgery—"

The woman decidedly did not look good. Steinman, a tall, graying surgeon, examined her swiftly but carefully. "Who knows what she may have broken loose? They shoved a proctoscope up her, they shoved barium up her, but not one responsible doctor even saw her—*oi, oi, oi*."

He got as much history as he could from the woman, got her quieted down a little, convinced her that she was not bleeding to death right then and there and then walked out of the room shaking his head. "This is insane," he said. "Whatever's going on in there, I've got to open her up and stop it." He turned to the G-2. "Get the OR crew moving—crash basis. Then get me Dr. Halar on the phone. He operated on this woman the last time, and I'm going to need him."

"Uh, I don't think Dr. Halar's on call," the G-2 said.

"I don't care if he's in China," Steinman said furiously. "I want Dr. Halar here, and I want him *now*. If you have to go to China to get him, go to China, but *move!* We'll be damned lucky not to end up with a corpse in bed in another thirty minutes!"

They didn't end up with a corpse in bed. Dan Halar, the surgeon who had done both of her previous colon resections, arrived quickly; he knew bad trouble when it kicked him in the head and didn't fool around selecting his socks. In the OR the two surgeons together stemmed the bleeding. A branch of the mesenteric artery had been eroded through from the disease, and another segment of colon had to be removed to stop the bleeding at four o'clock in the morning. Without any adequate assessment of the state of her colitis before the surgery, nor any opportunity really to quiet this newest attack, Mrs. Swedman was virtually certain to have recurrent trouble later, and Dr. Dan Halar and Dr. Avram Steinman and Dr. Ed Millikan and everybody else knew it. But at least Mrs. Swedman wasn't dead. She stayed in the hospital, with her restive and angry husband by her side, just long enough to be able to get up on her feet without falling over on her face again. Then she signed out of the hospital against medical advice, and without a single word to the army of Clinic doctors who were now in intensely close attendance upon her she and her husband went home to their farm in Faribault.

It was not the last the Mayo Clinic was to hear of the Swedmans, however. Already angry beyond words, Mr. Swedman—normally a hard-working, phlegmatic, third-generation Swedish-American farmer—was infuriated to receive a huge bill for ten days' hospitalization in Rochester Methodist Hospital and what seemed an especially insulting bill from the Mayo Clinic itemizing charges for professional services, emergency services, surgery and so forth. When he threw these bills in the wastebasket with a bit of pungent language, he subsequently received further communication from the two institutions urging him to make arrangements for payment at his earliest convenience.

Mr. Swedman was not a rich man, but like many other hard-working, phlegmatic, third-generation Swedish-American farmers in southern Minnesota, he had a little money tucked away under his mattress. Quite a bit of money, as a matter of fact. All the money he needed to hire the services of a hungry-eyed young attorney in Faribault who could recognize a live medical court case when it came walking down the pike. The next the Mayo Clinic and Rochester Methodist Hospital heard from Mr. and Mrs. Swedman, both institutions plus some seventeen assorted individual doctors (including Dr. Sandleman, who returned from his tour of the Rhine to find quite a number of angry colleagues waiting for him) learned that they were all, individually and collectively, being sued for $5.5 million on the basis of a bill of particulars some 123 items long. Not the least notable among them were such items as medical and surgical negligence and bald malpractice.

9

Rochester, Minnesota / *1895-1905*

In the past, books have been written about the "glory days of logging" in the late 1800s, when the hungry logging companies, having shaved off the northern Midwest forests bare as a pig's back, sent their logging crews to the Pacific Northwest with their long double-handled crosscut saws and their steam-driven donkey engines to take down the great ten- and twelve-foot-diameter Douglas fir trees as if there were no end to the supply. Others have written about the "glory days of railroading" after the Civil War, when the great transcontinental lines were opened and steel was laid from one end of this booming industrial country to the other and the robber barons like old Dr. Mayo's friend Jim Hill grew rich beyond belief from their spoils.

One could also speak of the "glory days of surgery" that blossomed in the civilized world in the twenty-year period between 1890 and 1910—a time when an exciting and vastly important new medical craft at last came fully into its own, a craft without which the treatment of human illness as we understand it today would be completely unthinkable.

During those years many ideas suddenly joined, and the whole was greater than any of its parts. Great men walked the land of medicine. There were Pasteur and Koch and the other great pioneer microbe hunters with their bacteria. There was Lister with his antiseptic surgery. There were

Morton and Crawford and others with their techniques for anesthesia. There was Rudolph Virchow and his great German school of microscopic pathology which led the way in discovering what diseased tissue was, what surgeons were actually operating on. And there were the surgeons themselves, all over the world, pushing back the barriers step by step, trying new things, bold things, unheard-of things, more and more confident that most of their patients would survive and that some of them, bless God, might actually benefit.

By 1890 Lister's techniques were being used carefully and properly almost everywhere that good surgery was being practiced. In fact, Lister's techniques were fast becoming old-fashioned. His idea was *antisepsis*—keeping everything around the patient as free of bacteria as possible. But surgeons soon evolved the even more logical concept of *asepsis—no bacteria at all* anywhere near the patient. This became possible with the development of steam boilers and autoclaves in which surgical drapes, instruments, gowns, masks and caps were not merely cleaned in a solution, which left some bacteria alive, but were actually sterilized, destroying *all* bacteria.

One great pioneer surgeon of the time was William Halsted at Johns Hopkins in Baltimore, who introduced a whole host of measures to prevent any possibility of infecting surgical patients in his operating room. Realizing that bacteria might survive under the fingernails or in the creases of the skin of the surgeon's hands, no matter how well they were scrubbed, Halsted tried using sterilized white cotton gloves during his operations but found them dreadfully sticky and messy to work with. By sheerest chance it happened that one of his operating-room nurses was suffering a severe skin outbreak on her hands from repeated immersion in strong antiseptic solutions and had started wearing a pair of thin sterilized rubber gloves to protect herself and still maintain antisepsis. Halsted was so intrigued by the idea that he had similar gloves manufactured for himself—and liked them. Soon other surgeons were also wearing sterilized rubber gloves for surgery—and the infection rate went down.

It was in exactly such stumbling fashion that other vital

innovations came about and real asepsis in the operating room became an achievable goal. The end result was that very soon the whole question of surgical infection became a matter of minor concern, even in very extensive surgical procedures. At the same time, pain disappeared as a barrier with the development of really good general anesthesias. In addition, the appearance of trained anesthesiologists, whether doctors or nurses, led to smoother, cleaner operating techniques. Nor was general anesthesia any longer the only thing available, quite literally knocking the patient unconscious no matter how large or small the surgical procedure. Cocaine, for example, was found capable of numbing a localized area of the body to provide local anesthesia without affecting the consciousness. One of the earliest proponents of cocaine was one Sigmund Freud of Vienna, who thought the stuff was grand and became quite actively habituated before its unpleasant properties became known. Halsted himself, in Baltimore, was so intrigued with the drug and did so much self-experimentation with its use as a regional anesthetic that he became almost disastrously habituated and had to interrupt a marvelously productive surgical career for some years before he could shake himself loose from it and come back to resume his work.

All in all, surgery was entering a period in which more and more surgeons began exploring what surgery could accomplish, exactly, with fewer and fewer disastrous results. Procedures were attempted that had never before been thought possible. True, sometimes the exploring was pushed too far too fast, and the period was strewn with corpses—but the corpses became fewer and fewer. If nothing else, such experimentation taught surgeons what they could *not* get away with as well as what they could.

Understandably, the surgeons who pioneered in this work fired the imagination of the world and became the rich, famous and glamorous figures in medicine. And because the Mayo brothers were extremely skillful surgeons with remarkably good medical and surgical judgment, they rose during this period to the top ranks of the rich, famous and glamorous. Will Mayo's comment some ten years before, as a graduate fresh from medical school, that he intended to stay in Rochester and become the greatest surgeon in the world, may have sounded silly and arrogant at the time—but by the year 1900 it seemed entirely possible.

Beginning about 1891, the two Mayo brothers were making regular study trips, each taking a month or so a year for intensive observation of the work of other surgeons. Since there were two of them, one was always at home keeping the store while the other was off and away. They didn't have to worry about their practice dwindling while they were gone. This worked especially well because, in those early days, Will and Charlie worked pretty much interchangeably. They both did the same procedures equally well and, when they were together in Rochester, often worked together in the same operating room, one operating, the other assisting.

Thus, during the 1890s, one or the other became familiar with the work of many leading surgeons in the East—Charles McBurney, another one who pioneered the treatment of acute appendicitis; Robert Abbe; William T. Bull; Robert Weir. They became acquainted with Joseph Price of Philadelphia, Christian Singer of Chicago, Nicholas Senn and John B. Murphy, one of the pioneers in bowel surgery. Will Mayo became especially close friends with another young surgeon, Albert Ochsner of Chicago, a friendship and friendly rivalry that was to persist for a lifetime. In 1894 Will met Dr. William Osler in Baltimore at Johns Hopkins and later, on a trip abroad, met Dr. Harvey Cushing, one of the all-time great neurosurgeons.

Always the brothers came home and applied what they learned—and often innovated and added on. For example, on a learning excursion to Boston in 1898, Will Mayo observed Dr. Maurice Richardson and Dr. Samuel Mixter doing never-before-heard-of operations on the stomach. Will Mayo saw what they were doing, figured out how the problems they were having could be solved and then set about improving when he got back home. Four years later, in 1902, these same Boston surgeons asked Will Mayo to come to Boston from Rochester to tell *them* how to do what *he* was doing in stomach surgery.

For all their interest in surgery during this time, the Mayo brothers were still very much general practitioners, with more and more of the burden of the large Rochester practice falling on their shoulders as their father grew older and less active. But surgery was more and more their special interest. To increase their opportunities to see surgical patients, they set up a volunteer surgical service at the State Hospital for the Insane in Rochester and in a similar hospital ninety miles to the west in St. Peter. They provided their services free of charge and reputedly continued for years after their need for extra experience had passed.

Bit by bit their surgical knowledge increased, as did the quality of the surgery they were doing. They recognized the critical difference between antisepsis and asepsis very early and were among the first surgeons in the country to install a sterilizer for surgical packs and instruments and to begin using Halsted's rubber gloves for every surgical procedure. Inevitably, they began to specialize between themselves: Will started doing most of the abdominal and gynecological surgery, while Charlie took over eye, ear, nose and throat surgery, bone and joint surgery, neurosurgery and surgery of the neck and thyroid.

For all their enthusiasm, they seemed to exercise good judgment as well. They were sensitive to the complaints of many doctors who thought that surgeons were going operation-crazy, especially as evidenced by the popularity of appendectomies that were now being done for practically any bellyache. The Mayos were more cautious, performing a total of only twelve appendectomies in the year 1895—but once convinced of the importance of early surgery for the disease, they began doing more and more—186 during the year 1900 and over a thousand in the year 1905. Other statistics testify to the growth of their work: In 1890 Will did his first operation for gallstones, merely removing the stones and inserting a drain. In 1900 he did seventy-five gall-bladder removals and 324 in 1905. In 1893 the brothers performed thirty-nine hernia repairs between them; by 1905 they were averaging 300 a year. They were also doing multitudes of other kinds of operations during this period, most notably surgery for cancers of internal organs such as the stomach. Indeed, the Mayos were among the country's leaders in recognizing that early cancer could be cured by surgery in many cases.

As the brothers' work and reputation flourished during this period, St. Mary's Hospital flourished along with them. During the first three and a half years of the hospital's operation the Mayos did fifty-four abdominal operations there. In 1900 alone they did 612 and in 1905, 2,157.

Even granting the developing skill and reputation of the Mayos, one still has to ask: *Where did all the patients come from?* There is no single, clear-cut answer. Partly, of course, patients came because of the expanding usefulness of surgery. Part of the Mayos' success was undoubtedly due to the time in which they entered their profession. Medicine was emerging at last from a period centuries long in which doctors really couldn't do very much about anything and patients who became ill either died or remained ill for decades. Here, the word suddenly got around, were *doctors who could do something,* and there was an enormous reservoir of long-standing illness in the countryside surrounding Rochester.

What was more, these were not men to sit back placidly and wait for work to drop into their laps. They were go-getters of a particularly aggressive sort, and it was this very aggressiveness that not only built their practice and reputations but also brought them the resentment and censure of other physicians that were to plague them for the rest of their lives. Certainly they did nothing to limit the spread of their reputations by word of mouth throughout the northern Midwest. They didn't precisely chase their patients, but they didn't mind in the least going to where a patient was if some surgeon in an outlying area called them for help, rather than making the patient come to Rochester.

Later, of course, these same patients and their doctors came back for further help and referred new patients to Rochester as well. As the railroads went through, people who were going out to the Dakotas and Wyoming where there was virtually no medical care at all would come back to Rochester when they became ill—and there was more and more surgery for the Mayo brothers to do. They did not, however, "discover" surgery to be done when surgery wasn't really called for, as some have contended. These men may have been almost indecently eager to operate and possibly over-certain of their correctness in urging a surgical patient to submit to the knife—but at least, by all accounts, they were honest to their own principles, truly convinced that what they were doing was right and sincerely concerned about their patients' welfare. In short, they were not hawking phony wares; they were simply very sharp at recognizing surgical disease when they saw it and were never reluctant to follow it up where they thought it might exist.

For example, among many other duties, Will accepted appointment as District Surgeon for the Minnesota and Dakota Divisions of the Chicago and Northwestern Railroad—and soon railroad people were coming to Rochester from places such as Omaha, LaCrosse and Dubuque. By the mid-1890s people were flocking into St. Mary's Hospital from Illinois, Kansas, Missouri, Nebraska, the Dakotas, Montana, New York and Ohio, as well as the more neighboring Iowa and Wisconsin.

This was also a period of great prosperity in Minnesota, with booming industries in timber, iron mining and flour milling. The population of the town of Duluth increased from 3,000 to 33,000 people in ten years, and as prosperity sifted down to the middle- and lower-class people in Minnesota, it became possible to go to Rochester for surgery when they needed it. True, Minneapolis and St. Paul also developed into an active surgical center at this time—but that was *not* the center that developed the international reputation. Skillful as the individual surgeons may have been in those cities to the north, surgical practice there was a dog-eat-dog affair. Somehow the close partnership and working team formed by the Mayos in Rochester, well isolated from nearby competitors, created a difference in attitude, ambiance and patient loyalty that made all the difference in the world.

The brothers settled in. In April 1893 Charlie married Edith Graham, daughter of a local pharmacist and a woman who had been serving the Mayos in their practice as an anesthetist, office nurse, general bookkeeper and secretary. Will had married Hattie Damon back in 1884, daughter of one of the pioneer residents of Rochester. She had borne him a daughter, Carrie, in 1887 and a son in August 1889, a fact that must have filled both father and grandfather with dreams of yet a third generation of Mayo doctors in Rochester—but the boy died at the age of three months and Will never fathered another. It remained for Charlie to produce sons in the Mayo family. In any event, both men established homes and family lives in Rochester. Ultimately Will was to build a large brick mansion on the top of a rise of land in southwestern Rochester—a house with a four-story tower at one corner reminiscent of the observatory tower his mother had had her husband build on the farm years before. Charlie, still remembering his childhood love of the farm, bought a large chunk of land south of the city and established a functioning farm there with a large rambling home built to house his growing family. The estate, which he named Mayowood, served him well for many decades as a home, retreat and recreational outlet alike; it still exists as a major point of historical interest in the Rochester area, with conducted tours for visitors two days a week.

By the early 1890s a watershed point was finally reached in the Mayos' practice. Old Dr. Mayo was becoming increasingly involved in state politics and local civic activies; he was growing eager to be free of practice obligations. The surgical practice was frankly getting out of hand for the brothers, with all the run-of-the-mill general practice obligations they also had to shoulder. More and more clearly they needed help and, for the first time ever, began looking outside the family to find it. In the neighboring town of Eyota, Minnesota, a fifty-year-old physician named Augustus W. Stinchfield had a longtime practice almost as large as the Mayos' and was held in high professional regard. Dr. Stinchfield was approached and agreed to come to Rochester to join as a partner in the Mayo brothers' practice. Arrangements were made to enlarge their downtown offices to make room for him.

He was the first.

The second was thirty-seven-year-old Dr. Christopher Graham, brother of the Edith Graham whom Charlie Mayo married and a man who, curiously enough, had started his professional career as a veterinarian trained at the University of Pennsylvania. He wasn't happy at it; he really wanted to be a doctor of human medicine, and the Mayos talked him into going back for the additional year necessary to gain a medical degree, on the promise that he could then come back and work with them. This he did and in 1893 became a second new partner in the practice.

It was planned that these men would relieve Will and Charlie of some of the enormous nonsurgical practice burden that was breaking their backs, and gradually many nonsurgical patients were shifted into the new doctors' hands. The Mayos, after all, were spending almost full time now operating at St. Mary's or handling surgical consultations, so it was up to the new partners to take the country calls, make extensive daily home rounds, perform much of the routine office patient work and deliver the babies.

Dr. Graham, for example, fell heir to most of the pregnancy cases and might have become the first real obstetrical specialist in the practice had he not gotten sidetracked in an interesting way. New diagnostic lab tests and methods were appearing on the horizon in medicine, and Kit Graham learned about some of these on his return to Pennsylvania. Laboratory studies of gastric juice, for example, were proving an important aid to the diagnosis of stomach ailments, so that a surgeon had a far better chance of telling exactly what was going on in a patient's stomach before he operated to find out. It made considerable difference whether a patient had a duodenal ulcer or a cancer of the stomach in order to plan what kind of operation to do.

Similarly, more sophisticated methods of urinalysis could provide the surgeon with a much better idea of what was happening in the kidney or urinary tract before surgery. Dr. Graham became fascinated with this kind of lab analysis, and of course it appealed mightily to Will and Charlie too. Soon Graham had rigged up a new clinical laboratory next to his examining room on the second floor of the Mayo offices, and the first steps were taken to provide the practice with up-to-date laboratory diagnosis and clinical pathology. When X rays appeared on the scene late in 1895, yet another powerful diagnostic tool became available. For three years the Mayos used another doctor's X-ray machine in Rochester, but in 1900 the brothers bought their own machine and—characteristically—improved its design to better serve their own needs.

Others joined the group, formally or informally, either as partners or as employees. Sister Joseph, acting as nurse in addition to hospital administrator, became a virtual first assistant in the operating room for both brothers. Dr. Gertrude Booker, recently graduated from the University of Minnesota, was chosen by Dr. Charles Mayo to take over the job of testing patients' eyes and fitting glasses. Dr. Melvin C. Millet came to help with diagnosis of urinary-tract problems and soon became master of the cystoscope, a device for direct examination of the inside of the bladder, as well as other clinical laboratory techniques, and Dr. Isabella Herb came to Rochester in 1899, recommended by Will's surgeon friend Dr. Albert Ochsner, to serve as Charlie's chief anesthetist. In addition, Dr. Henry Plummer joined the group, a strange and extraordinary man who was destined to make an indelible mark on the entire Mayo organization as years went by.

All these early additions to the group came specifically to handle aspects of the practice that Will and Charlie could no longer manage due to their preoccupation with surgery. The brothers were the Surgeons. In 1903, however, a striking departure occurred. A local man named Edward Starr Judd, after completing medical school at the University of Minnesota, had come back to St. Mary's Hospital as an intern, and for the first time the Mayo brothers considered taking on another surgeon as an associate. The man was skillful, gifted, untiring and thoroughly compatible with the brothers themselves. Thus in 1903 Dr. Judd was hired to work as Charlie Mayo's first assistant in surgery and to help see patients in the office. A year later he was appointed junior surgeon in the practice and ultimately became a full surgical partner in the group, the first ever.

With the practice growing, St. Mary's Hospital had to enlarge. A four-story addition was built in 1897, tacked onto the original building, to increase the size of the hospital to 154 beds. Those beds were full before the addition was finished, with patients having to wait for days for their surgery because there was no place to put them. In 1904 still another addition was built: an east wing of four stories providing a total of 175 beds, space for the surgeons to use for changing clothes or resting between procedures, two operating rooms, a sterilizing room and even a special lounge for the visiting doctors who were beginning to flock to Rochester to see for themselves what these Mayo brothers they'd heard about were doing.

New members in the group created problems, and policies had to be made to deal with them. For one thing, there was the question of money. At the beginning, when Will and Charlie were alone, there wasn't much money to speak of and the brothers had sort of an unwritten agreement about how it should be handled. They had a single bank account between them, each drew on it as he needed to, and neither made an accounting to anybody.

But now money was pouring in, more than either brother really needed for the comparatively simple way of life they had chosen for themselves. It didn't come from exorbitant fees or hardhearted business practices. By all accounts, both men were generous and compassionate in financial dealings with their patients. They charged no more than going rates for the surgery they were doing. The money rolled in because of the sheer volume of that surgery.

Both men worked hard and firmly believed that the patients who could pay for their surgery and other medical care jolly well ought to—but they didn't want patients hurting on account of medical costs, either, and they treated many patients for nothing at all. Ultimately certain policies they had always followed more or less informally were formally codified for themselves and their associates. They would charge nothing for their services to other doctors, nurses, clergymen or their dependents. They would set standard fees for those who were able to pay and charge others according to what they *could* pay. On the other hand, they would not let their fees become an economic burden if they could help it. Perhaps most important of all, they doggedly regarded money and medical care as two different things. Everybody got the same quality care, no matter what they were paying. Today, with the hordes of people who regard free medical care as their natural birthright and with many doctors unhappy with six-figure incomes, it all sounds faintly naïve and Boy Scoutish and not very realistic, but in those days it made a simple, generous kind of grass-roots sense—and it *worked*.

As the money came in, it had to be used. Much of the Mayos' money was invested, better and better as they found sound-minded business people to advise them. The doctors joining them were paid well, not exactly handsomely but enough to provide a decent living. They also received funds for travel and study to improve their skills. Nor were the Mayos niggardly in providing the equipment and facilities needed for each associate to practice the best quality of medicine he could. When some new advancement occurred, some new diagnostic technique, some new machine, instrument or device, the money was available.

Early on, when a small but unpleasant battle arose over one point of financial policy, the Mayos resolved it in characteristic fashion. The question was: What part of the value of the growing practice, its equipment and its facilities, was to be the personal, individual property of any given staff doctor if he were to resign or to die?

The brothers had never given it a thought, but faced with the problem, they discussed it and came up with an answer: none. On resignation, retirement or death a partner or his estate would be entitled to a sum of money equal to his last year's salary, and beyond that the surviving partners would have no further obligation to him. To make it stick, Will Mayo had this edict written up by a lawyer as a formal contract and presented it to each associate for signature. Certain of them thought it was unfair, and balked, and stalled, and refused to sign. Will Mayo took all the delay he cared to put up with, and then laid it out flat on the table: Sign now, or get out and we'll just dissolve this partnership. One way or the other, whatever you like, but do it *now*. The balkers signed. Unfair? Maybe. Ruthless? Some surely thought so. But also, perhaps, almost incredibly farsighted—for without that agreement the group would almost certainly have fallen apart over the issue sooner or later.

Bit by bit, members of the group gravitated into their natural roles. Drs. Stinchfield and Graham became the diagnosticians but almost entirely *surgical* diagnosticians; the medical side of the practice was definitely getting short shrift. Will and Charlie Mayo and the upcoming Starr Judd were full-time surgeons. Henry Plummer took over the clinical laboratory and X-ray diagnosis but spent time doing other strange things as well. One of his early projects, for example, was a systematic, painstaking scientific study of thyroid disease—a task that fit hand in glove with Charlie Mayo's increasing interest in thyroid surgery. Plummer also worked to design systems and devices to simplify the group's efforts in seeing patients, allowing them to spend more time practicing medicine and waste less time on nonsense. One such device was a system of colored signals, like railroad flags, outside examining rooms, so doctors would know at a glance which patients they were to see in which rooms. Plummer also reorganized the patient record system and later became a major architectural designer for the group.

Meanwhile, as patients poured into Rochester, hotels and roominghouses began to flourish to provide lodging for the Mayos' patients. Will and Charlie must have seen the investment opportunities that were clearly present in such ventures, but they decided not to participate. Instead they encouraged men such as young John Kahler, son of an old-time hotelkeeper, to put the old Cook House, a decrepit Rochester landmark, back on its feet and turn it into a forty-five-room hotel. Boardinghouses flourished and restaurants appeared. Rochester was still a small country town in 1900, with a population of around 5,000 to 6,000 people, but remarkable things were happening there. The streets were being paved, a park was being developed with the help of Mayo dollars, and the Mayo brothers were looking farther afield for new people to join them as the practice kept growing one step ahead of their capacity to handle it.

Somewhere along the line in 1905 or 1906 a term appeared describing this group of doctors in Rochester, with their offices in a downtown building and their close working relationship with St. Mary's Hospital. Apparently it arose not from patients but from doctors discussing their visits to the Mayos' operating rooms. They began speaking of this remarkable group practice in southern Minnesota as "the Mayo brothers' clinic at St. Mary's Hospital" or just "the Mayos' Clinic."

The name stuck.

10
Rochester,
Minnesota / *June 1979*

It was late on Thursday afternoon when Mary Manetti Petri stood by a window in a visitors' lounge in St. Mary's Hospital and stared out at the busy construction of the New Addition currently in progress. A violent thunderstorm had come up over the city an hour or so before, chilling Mary, since she had always associated thunderstorms with disaster for as long as she could remember. Now the storm was disappearing to the west, however, and sunlight was filtering through. There was no word, yet, of disaster from the place they had taken her husband, somewhere down in the bowels of this strangely homey and old-fashioned-seeming hospital. He had disappeared hours before into the maw of an elevator, with men and women in white and blue-green pajamas and caps, IV bottles swinging from poles attached to the stretcher, as though he were sick or something.

As though he were sick or something, indeed, she thought. Well, he *was* sick. She knew that all too well. Dr. O'Shaughnessy was a good, kind man, a pleasant sort of man, but he had not been joking when he had told them how very sick a man Giacomo Petri might be. Now they were in the process of finding out just how sick he really was, and it took forever and forever and forever.

She was filled with gloom, seriously thinking of leaving her post and going down to the street where hundreds of people seemed to be putting away umbrellas and struggling out of raincoats, down to go walking somewhere, anywhere, just to be doing something. But even as the thought formed the elevator near the lounge opened and Ian O'Shaughnessy stepped out, looking surprisingly fresh and chipper in his brightly checkered summer sport jacket and pale-blue slacks. "Well, Mrs. Petri," he said, "that stage of the journey is over."

"You've finished, then," she said. "And Jake?"

"Jake's doing fine," O'Shaughnessy said. "There were no problems at all. We had to worry you about them because they sometimes happen, and we still have to keep our fingers crossed another twenty-four hours against the outside chance that something still might happen. I don't think it will, but you had to know about that possibility too."

"I know," the woman said. "It would be truly horrible to think that nothing could happen and then have a trap door open under you. I guess it's better to know and to worry." She looked at the neurosurgeon. "But now you have to tell me what you learned from these—these angiograms and things."

"We learned a great deal. On that score, at least, the risk was very much worth it." He seemed reluctant to go on.

"And what did you learn?" she asked.

The man sighed. "First, we learned he has *not* yet had a major stroke, and that's good news, because if he had, it would limit us terribly, close doors to us that we really want open. It leaves us some options. Second, I'm virtually certain he has no brain tumor, no cancer, no brain abscess."

"Then what *does* he have?" Mary Petri asked.

"He has no functioning left internal carotid artery," Dr. O'Shaughnessy said.

"You'd better explain that to me, I think."

"I'll draw you a picture." He took out a pad and a pencil. "Normally the head receives its blood supply from two great arteries, the carotids, that come up from the heart, one on the left side of the neck, the other on the right. Up here at the base of the skull each carotid splits into an external and internal branch. Essentially, the left internal carotid feeds the left side of the brain the blood and oxygen it needs to work properly. The other internal carotid feeds the other side. Jake has a virtually total blockage of the internal carotid artery on the left. There's no blood going through it. None at all."

"But why not?"

"Because somehow it's gotten plugged up. It couldn't have happened suddenly, because if it had, it would have killed him, then and there. We know from our studies that he has a certain amount of atherosclerosis—a hardening and narrowing of arteries in various parts of his body. Partly this could be a function of his age, partly a function of his diet over the years, maybe partly a function of what he inherited from his mother and father—but the condition can lead to obstruction of certain vital arteries over the years. And at some point, eight or more months ago—perhaps years ago— this particular carotid artery began plugging up, a little at a time. I suspect he began having his symptoms when it was about two thirds blocked. They got worse as it plugged up more and more. Now it's completely shut."

"Then how does his brain get oxygen on that side?" Mary Petri asked.

"From the right internal carotid," Dr. O'Shaughnessy replied. "The unplugged one." He took the pad and pencil again. "Sometimes nature has a way of foreseeing trouble and protecting us against really bad emergencies. By extreme good fortune there happens to be a point down here at the base of the brain—" he scribbled a diagram— "where there's an interconnecting circle of arteries, a really complete circle. It's called the Circle of Willis, after some moldy old anatomist who first discovered it. Its job normally is to supply blood to the base of the brain and other structures in the immediate area—but it just happens to connect the right internal carotid system with the left."

"So blood can get through from one side to the other," Mary said.

"Exactly. Ordinarily, blood goes into this circle from both carotids. But when one carotid gets plugged below the level of the Circle of Willis—that is, nearer to the heart—then some of the blood from the right side can cross through the circle and go into the other carotid above the obstruction. That's why Jake hasn't been completely incapacitated by this thing, or even killed. With *some* blood getting over there, he's just barely been able to sneak by."

The woman sighed. "That's certainly what he's been doing," she said. "That's what he'll keep on doing, too, as long as he can. One thing about that man—he fights. He won't quit."

"Well, he might well keep sneaking by for a while, maybe for months or even years, if he cuts back on everything. But meanwhile, nerve cells in that starving side of his brain are dying, one by one. Lots of them must already be destroyed. A lot more are in the process of going unless they get more blood very soon. In other words, we can't count on his staying the way he is now. He's going to get progressively worse. How fast or how much worse I don't know—but worse. In addition, if something were to happen to plug up that *right* internal carotid, he's had it. That would not be a stroke from which he might recover. It'd all be over in a hurry."

"So he's walking a tightrope," Mary Petri said. "It's just a question of how soon he falls off. And there's *nothing* to be done?"

"You're rushing me," Dr. O'Shaughnessy said. He walked over to the window, looked out across the green park, watched a huge Cadillac from Missouri down below block up traffic in both directions as it tried to make a U-turn in front of the hospital. "I've been telling you where things are as of today, what's already happened and what Jake's chances are if he *doesn't* have treatment. The fact is, knowing what we do now, there *is* something to be done. It's extremely difficult to do and carries very real risks, but when it works it can do remarkable things. The trick is to get more blood into the left internal carotid artery or one of its branches *above* the blockage—not just a little blood but *lots* of it, to start feeding that starving brain tissue again.

"What we do, essentially, is look for another artery, one with plenty of blood going through it, but one that he can spare, like one of the big arteries feeding the scalp, for example. Then we make a hole in his skull and plug that scalp artery directly into a branch of the left internal carotid above the obstruction—and suddenly he's got blood again where he needs it. This connection of arteries is an extremely delicate job, using the tiniest imaginable sutures; in fact, we have to do it under a microscope. At the same time, we monitor his brain function constantly throughout the procedure, as well as heart function and blood pressure, so we know if something's going wrong. Throughout the whole thing, I work hand in glove with a vascular surgeon. It takes both of us, and then some."

"But it works," Mary Petri said.

"Most times it works. If we can find suitable arteries to use, and if we can get a good connection with our microsurgery, and if the vessels don't plug up or send blood clots to the lung, and if the connection doesn't tear loose, we can usually win. We can't restore dead nerve cells, but the brain has a vast surplus of nerve cells. We can hope to reverse the injury to nerve cells that are merely damaged but not quite dead. This means there can be recovery of lost function, sometimes very rapid, dramatic recovery, sometimes a slower process over a period of months. And at the same time, we can hope to protect against further brain-cell destruction."

"You spoke about risks," the woman said. "The other day when you talked about risks we didn't really pay too much attention. We obviously had to know what was wrong with Jake. But now I guess we really do have to pay attention. As Jake would say, what are the percentages?"

"They're not as good as we'd like," Dr. O'Shaughnessy said, "but they're not all that bad, either. We've done about a hundred and ten of these procedures here so far. Among our patients, somewhere between four and five percent have died, either during the surgery or within the first seventy-two hours postoperatively. Sixteen percent or so survived, all right, but just didn't show any measurable improvement. Another two percent survived the surgery but ended up *worse* then they were before, for various reasons. That leaves about seventy-eight percent who not only survived the surgery but did show real, measurable, identifiable improvement. In those cases the improvement has ranged all the way from the barely noticeable to the very striking. Unfortunately, there's no guessing just where within that range any given patient is going to fall."

"And how long does this improvement last?"

The surgeon spread his hands. "We're dealing with a dynamic, ever-changing life process, and our ability to do this kind of surgery at all is so very new we can't yet talk in terms of five or ten or twenty years. We can only talk about winning a year at a time, and watching, and keeping records, and seeing what happens."

"And what about alternatives to the surgery? *Are* there any alternatives?"

"The best alternative would be treatment with blood-thinning agents to cut down the tendency toward further blood clotting. Actually, old Dr. Johnson in Fargo was right on target with his aspirin—we use it here, and it helps. Other drugs do too. But none of them opens up a closed artery. None dissolves an obstruction, and none stops the progressive hardening and narrowing of arteries."

"I see." Mary looked up at the neurosurgeon. "When do you think this should be done, if Jake wants to go ahead?"

"The sooner the better," Dr. O'Shaughnessy said, "once we're completely satisfied that he's recovered from the arteriogram. Monday morning would be perfect."

Mary Petri nodded and rose to leave, retrieving her handbag. She turned to the little neurosurgeon and took his hand in both of hers. "I can't thank you enough for what you've already done," she said. "The time you've spent and the care you've taken to help us understand. Of course, Jake is the one who'll have to decide now. I think I know his answer. He's always been a bit of a gambler, but I can't decide this for him."

"Of course you can't," the doctor said. "Just talk it over together, that's all. I'll see you both later on this evening, in case you have other questions, and then again tomorrow morning. Then we can see."

Ian O'Shaughnessy headed on down the elevator and out

to his car. With the facility of long practice and skill, a true survival quality for neurosurgeons, he was already erasing from his mind, for the present, the tricky decision the Petris had to face and was focusing on the seven or eight patients he still had to see at the Clinic that day. One, he feared, was going to be a nightmare: a well-known woman novelist with an acoustic neuroma that must have been growing in her skull for at least fifteen years. He shuddered as he thought of it and turned his car into the traffic on 2nd Street S.W.

There is possibly no harder task for a writer than to describe a medical research laboratory accurately and make it sound impressive. No matter what exciting findings may emerge from such places, the labs themselves always just seem messy. Nobel Prize winners work in labs that look like rats' nests, with last year's gum wrappers scattered all over the floor.

Certainly John Porter, the small, weasel-faced young man who worked in the research administration office at Mayo Clinic, seemed highly apologetic about appearances as he whisked me along on a lightning tour of some of the research laboratories that cloudy, cool Friday morning. Some of the labs were in the old Medical Sciences Building, with its maze of narrow, tunnellike corridors, its polished floor tiles yellowing, the corridor walls painted an institutional beige color which had darkened to a sort of mud-brown. Other labs were in the upper stories of the spanking new Conrad Hilton Building, shiny and spotless and expensive-looking and—it seemed to me—surprisingly empty for a building which had supporting pillars emerging from the roof against the day when a few more stories might have to be added.

But old building or new, the labs themselves all looked much the same—cluttered with equipment, some in use, some temporarily retired and just sitting there, benches and stools and files, banks of incubators, piles of journals, and always the obligatory computer terminal occupying some prominent spot, as if to declare that without a computer terminal these days a research lab was really not a proper research lab at all. In many of the labs one could see people in stained white coats sitting on stools and sipping coffee out of plastic cups, intent on their quiet conversation, then stopping in mid-sentence and looking up as we walked by, as though we might possibly have overheard something. Other labs, with doors closed, carried the familiar yellow and blue three-spoke warning symbol and the sign: KEEP OUT, RADIOACTIVE MATERIALS, AUTHORIZED PERSONNEL ONLY. Corridor after corridor of labs, floor after floor of labs.

"But what do they all do?" I asked my guide, John Porter.

"Almost anything you could think of," he said. "Some of this is pure, basic, biomedical research—biochemistry, physiology, even anatomy. You'd think we'd already know everything there was to know about human anatomy by now, wouldn't you? After all, you can lay the cadaver open on the table and look at it and what more is there to find out? But you'd be wrong. At least two guys here have been trying for the last year to track down the microdetail of tiny veins draining the bowel. Seems ridiculous, but they think they can learn something new and useful about how cells from a colon cancer spread to the liver. Right now they're studying dogs, using dyes and radioactive tracers. Other people are studying how to convert certain triglyceride molecules into slightly different ones, or how to take a hormone molecule apart and figure out how it carries its message, or how to knock a 'killer radical' off one of the cell poisons they use against cancer so it won't be so likely to kill the patient along with the disease. None of this necessarily has any practical application at this point, but then that's not necessarily what they're here for."

"Surely they must do *some* practical research," I broke in.

"Oh, my, yes. Some are doing very practical work indeed—running controlled animal tests on new drugs so we can get FDA approval for human studies, for example. Or doing a slide-by-slide review of ten thousand surgical specimens from stomach cancer patients in order to work out a better way to stage the progress of the disease in a given patient and then run a computerized statistical analysis to see which of seven different surgical techniques for gastrectomy led to the longest patient survival in each of ten stages of cancer development. With all those variables, a study like that would have taken a man half a lifetime to complete twenty-five years ago. Now the only time-eater is reading the slides and programming the computer properly—and we may soon even have the computer screening the slides for us. There's one doctor and two assistants on that little project right now, and they expect to be ready to publish in a year."

Porter whisked me around a corner and into an elevator going up. We stepped off into a dank little corner in the old building. "Actually," he said, "the variety of research here covers the spectrum from one end to the other, and it's largely hassle-free. You take the average big tax-supported medical school–medical center–hospital institution, and everybody's scared all the time, begging for money, fighting for lab space, depending for their lifework on federal grants that may be cut off halfway through because the President gets nervous about inflation. Even when those people *get* their grant money, the university has its belly right up to the feed trough, taking half of the dollars right off the top. 'Administrative costs,' they call it—but if the guy finds he needs half a dozen extra test tubes he's got to write a ten-page justification in order to get them. Then, when one of his key technicians quits, he discovers that the university has frozen hiring in order to 'economize,' so he has to work short-handed for the next ten months. And if by chance he finds he can actually make do with *less* money than he got, he'd damned well better spend it anyway, because not a nickel of it can be carried over to next year, and the government will cut next year's grant because he didn't spend all of this year's. And finally, of course, he's got to spend about six months of his time every year getting his grant application written up for next year instead of doing his research. And if you think all this is a gross exaggeration, you just go talk to some of those poor bastards working in those settings and see what *they* say."

"I don't need to," I said. "I already know."

"Well, we have problems, too, but we don't have quite that much trouble. If a man wants to do research, he can get help from Mayo funds as well as federal grants. The lab space is here. If he needs help, we can hire him help. If he needs equipment, we buy it. Only about fifty-five percent of our research budget comes from federal grant money, and we don't take anywhere near the amounts off the top for 'administrative costs' that most places do. We don't *like* having to take government money—Will and Charlie Mayo would have had fits—and we have to hold the line tightly on new work, but some very expensive projects really demand federal help. Let's see if Sam Lundwall's in—he's involved in our big DSR project. One of the sharpest bioengineering minds in the country, Sam is."

We went around a corner to a cubbyhole office and found one of the sharpest bioengineering minds in the country sitting at his desk working on a crossword puzzle. Trained at the University of Uppsala in Sweden, Dr. Sam Lundwall looked barely old enough to be shaving. He was a tall, thin, blond young man wearing a pair of thick Coke-bottle glasses right out of the old Dr. Cyclops movies. Aside from the obligatory heaps of journals scattered around, most of his tiny lab-office was filled with a huge blackboard covered from top to bottom with mathematical symbols and equations written in such a scrawl that no human being could conceivably have read them.

Rather shyly, Dr. Lundwall told us about his project: the immense Dynamic Spatial Reconstructor now being assembled in the huge circular room upstairs. This device, when completed, would surround a patient's body with a battery of twenty-eight high-speed X-ray portals that would take up to 75,000 low-voltage X-ray pictures of the patient in the course of five seconds.

"After all," Lundwall said, "the organs we're trying to examine are dynamic, constantly moving systems. We put dye into a great blood vessel, it enters the heart, passes out to the lungs or out into the coronary arteries and dissipates. This all happens very fast. One X-ray picture shows us what is happening at a particular instant, but not the instant before or after. With this little beauty we're building we can follow the entire cycle from every imaginable angle for the space of five or six heartbeats. Then all that image data then goes into the computer and we come up with a three-dimensional hologram of the patient's functioning insides. It'll look a *little* bit like what I'm going to show you."

He led us down a darkened hallway to a bank of TV screens, dug a video tape out of a drawer and fed it into a machine. A moment later I was watching a fantastic display of a living, moving heart on the screen, rotating as if seen in three dimensions, showing the circulation of blood actually moving *through* the coronary arteries. At one point the heart image split open to reveal the interior, the valves opening and closing with each heartbeat. "We did this one on a dog," Dr. Lundwall said. "There now, you can see where we tied off the left anterior coronary. "No circulation there, now, and you can see the difference in density in the infarcted area of the heart fed by that artery Of course we know the left anterior coronary is the bad one for humans, but you need to know what you've got in order to do an efficient job of bypassing a block there."

He snapped off the film. "Now, this film is only *simulated* Three-D, and it's terribly limited. To make it we had to jury-rig a little test machine with only five small X-ray portals, and we didn't have the firing of the X rays mechanized; we had to fire them off manually. And we had to rotate the subject instead of the machine, and it was a real mess. The computer smoothed off some of the rough edges with image enhancement, but we still don't know if we're seeing what actually happened or something that the computer made up. But with that big beauty upstairs with twenty-eight high-speed X-ray portals and everything automatic and the big computer—now *that's* going to be something else. Meanwhile, Dr. Choppin over in the Clinic is already using our little five-unit machine to try to pinpoint lung cancers, even tiny ones, far earlier than usual."

Back in his office, we talked a bit more, and then Dr. Lundwall began edging back toward his crossword puzzle, so we excused ourselves. Porter guided me back to the Conrad

Hilton Building, where we took an elevator up to the top floor. He paused by a door and said, "Here, this may give you a bit of a jolt."

He pulled open the door and ushered me in. A wave of rank animal odor swept over me as I stepped through the portal, so strong it made my eyes water, and the din that arose at our appearance was almost deafening. We were in a huge room crammed from floor to ceiling with bank upon bank of cages, large and small, each containing an almost humanlike creature. There were spider monkeys, gibbons, macaques, rhesus monkeys, half a dozen exceedingly noisy chimpanzees, including one female nursing an almost naked bug-eyed baby. A baboon with hideous facial markings and hideous-looking teeth charged me from the far side of his cage with an earsplitting scream and began gnawing viciously at the wire as if he were coming right through. In another cage a huge brown monkey hung by its tail from a bar and opened one yellow eye as I walked past, then closed it again and reached up to scratch its belly.

"The primate room," John Porter explained. "These animals are just the ones that are actively needed right now. The dog room and cat room are farther down the hall. We have more, of course, out on the Farm—that's what we call our extended animal facility a few miles south of town. And we keep other animals out there too—chickens, ducks, pigs, calves. Somebody was even doing blood-pressure studies on a donkey, I think."

He glanced at his watch and shrugged apologetically. "I'm afraid I have to get on to a meeting," he said. "I'll take you back down to Desk C and you can find your way from there. Over all, the research program is just one leg of the 'three-legged stool' concept that makes Mayo Clinic what it is today. Patient care, of course, is the leg of the stool you think of first, obviously the biggest and most familiar aspect. Research is the second leg, equally important, in its way, even if it's less in the public eye. Medical teaching is the third leg—the whole program for interns and residents and Fellows, graduate training for doctors after they finish medical school, and now the new Mayo Medical School to take prospective doctors through their basic medical training as well. And it all built up from the basic grand scheme Will and Charlie Mayo got rolling so many years ago. They were visionaries, those men, as well as doctors, believe me. They were whole decades ahead of their time—which is why the Mayo Clinic is here today."

On Friday morning Dr. Howard Norgaard parked his car at St. Mary's and paused for a moment to survey the long, sprawling façade of the hospital. It had grown like a nautilus, a chunk at a time, and one could identify the different chunks, each varying slightly from the rest in the architectural styling, the decorative features, the darkness or lightness of the brick and stone, stretching out more than two city blocks along 2nd Street S.W. Now, the newest addition was well under way. More bed space was needed, more offices and labs and auxiliary space, new operating rooms— but this time things were planned quite differently. Always before, new additions had been financed privately, bought and paid for privately. But the $55 million project now under construction was just too big a bite for the hospital to swallow on a private basis. For the first time, municipal bonds had been issued by the City of Rochester to finance the project. Ground-breaking took place September 30, 1977, with completion expected early in 1980. *And so it grows*, Norgaard reflected. *And soon we'll need some of Henry Plummer's vacuum tubes to hurl doctors from one end of the place to another.*

When he met his crew for morning rounds Norgaard said, "Let's see Manuela first" and headed off toward the cardiac intensive-care unit.

"Uh, Dr. Norgaard, I'm afraid she's not there any more," Buzz Turnbull said gloomily.

"What do you mean, she's not there?"

The young doctor barely suppressed his grin. "Dr. Hornby thought she needed a change of scene, needed all those tubes pulled out. So he sent her up to the pediatric floor this morning to see how she gets along."

"But what about the supports?"

"He thinks she doesn't need them. The cardiac monitor

has been stable for two days now—that arrhythmia she had stopped all of a sudden and never recurred. She's completely afebrile and manages to get around on her feet just fine with support from a nurse. And she's been tolerating fluids by mouth and a soft diet for twenty-four hours, so she doesn't need IVs. Mostly, Charlie thought, what she really needs is visitors like her parents and somebody to play with."

"This I've got to see," Norgaard said.

Compared to the nightmarish science-fiction setting of the cardiac intensive-care unit, the pediatric floor was like a bright and airy children's playground. The corridors and rooms of the children's section were filled with cheerful color, the various rooms labeled in large letters with saucy titles the children themselves had thought up to identify them. The examination room had SHOW AND TELL painted diagonally across the door, and the head nurse's office sported the label BOSS LADY. The Boss Lady herself came out to join them and took them down to Manuela's sunny room—but the girl was not there. Auxiliary support equipment was standing by but obviously not in use. "She may be down in the game room," the nurse said. "Of course she has a special with her around the clock."

Manuela was in an alcove marked ROMPER ROOM, sitting with her mother working on a jigsaw puzzle and chattering away in Spanish. As they approached, Dr. Norgaard—almost unbelieving—heard a tinkle of laughter.

God, he thought, *you leave town for twenty-four hours and they cure themselves. I should go to more conferences in Chicago.*

He could hardly believe the transformation in the girl. Gone were the sallow, yellow complexion, the blue circles under the eyes and the purple lips; she was *pink*, with a sparkle in her eye and animation in her face he had never seen before. She was still a spindly little scarecrow with black-and-blue arms, still slow and cautious in her movements, but no longer wincing with every breath. Before he had left for his one-day trip to Chicago she had looked like a breathing corpse with the cold, waxy yellow aspect of death about her; now she looked like a sick little girl who was very rapidly getting better.

She was laughing again as he walked into the room. Then she saw him, and her face fell. He grinned at her. "I see you've changed rooms," he said.

"*Sí*. Dr. Hornby's nice to me."

"And it doesn't hurt to laugh now."

"Oh yes it does," she said quickly. "But not so much." She sat still, tolerated his examination of her chest with his stethoscope. She looked up at him sullenly. "You going to send me back to that awful place?"

Her mother began to shush her in Spanish, but Norgaard flashed her a warning. "You mean where all the tubes and hoses and machines are? Well, I don't know. It all depends. Are you still so mad at me?"

Suddenly the girl's eyes were more sly than angry. "Maybe not *quite*," she said.

Dr. Norgaard leaned over and studied the picture puzzle very carefully. "How do I know you're not mad?" he asked. "Maybe you're just saying it."

Manuela glanced quickly at her mother, then leaned over with a giggle and kissed him on the cheek. "There!" she said, as if relations now were completely repaired. "We have, the way you say, kissed and made up."

Howard Norgaard controlled himself like iron until he was out of the room and halfway down the corridor toward the elevator. Then, without warning, he stopped and seized Buzz Turnbull in an enormous bear hug, lifting him off his feet and whirling him around, pounding him on the back. "By God, Buzz, we've made it, do you realize that? We've made it!"

"You mean Manuela has made it," the other one said, back on his feet once more.

"It's the same thing," Howard Norgaard said. "I tell you for true, man, it's exactly the same thing."

The young man sitting across from me in one of the leather-upholstered chairs in the cozy lounge of the Student Center later that morning did not precisely reflect the Mayo image that I had grown accustomed to seeing in Rochester. His hair tumbled in ringlets down to his shoulders. A straggly beard concealed most of his face. He wore grubby tennis shoes with the toes worn through, threadbare blue jeans and a pale-blue T-shirt bearing the image of a fat Oriental Buddha with one finger upraised in instruction and the words YUCK FOO! inscribed in large yellow letters underneath. The girl in the other chair looked even less Mayoish, if possible—a rather blowsy young woman with large nipples thrusting vigorously at her thin jersey blouse and the words HANDS OFF embroidered, amidst flowers and marijuana leaves, across the seat of her dungarees. Hardly the Mayo image, yet both these young people were likely to carry the name and prestige of the Mayo Clinic with them throughout the rest of their professional careers. Larry Silverman of New York City would soon be a junior in the Mayo Medical School, class of 1981. Hazel Wasnowski from Gary, Indiana, would be a sophomore in the same school, class of 1982.

Both of them looked exceedingly sleepy, and probably they were; both had been studying for final exams, and I was very lucky to corner them at all. But both seemed proud of the medical school they were attending and happy to talk about its programs. The Mayo Medical School was the newest such institution in the country, admitting its first class in 1972 and graduating it in 1976. It was also one of the smallest such schools in the country, with just forty seats in the freshman class, a total of 160 in the entire school—"but they plan to have more, once they get better organized," Larry said. The student body seemed to be a comfortable, close-knit group, surprisingly ecumenical, with thirty-nine female students, seven blacks, two Orientals, one Chicano and one Amerindian.

The school had been established partly as a result of earlier governmental pressures on the medical establishment to enlarge training facilities for physicians. Even more, it had been the final realization of the Mayo brothers' old, original dream: to establish a great center in Rochester for the education and training of physicians, even, eventually, down to the undergraduate medical-school level. "Certainly the clinical facilities were here," Hazel said. "Almost two thousand hospital inpatients and tens of thousands of outpatients in the Clinic; some of the top-ranking physicians in the country on the Clinic staff and a lot of them eager to teach. Of course they had to arrange lab facilities for student teaching, which they didn't have, and make some other adjustments, but it wasn't too big a reach when they finally decided to do it."

I asked the two about their programs of study. It bore scant resemblance to my own medical-school training twenty-five years before, when students spent the first two full years studying nothing but the basic laboratory sciences, dissecting cadavers, studying physiology, pathology, micro-anatomy, neuroanatomy and biochemistry, spending days and months behind reagent bottles in laboratories, peering through microscopes and hardly ever seeing a living patient until the beginning of the third year. But medical schools don't do it that way any more, and the Mayo Medical School was very much in tune with the times.

"We do it all by systems now," Larry said. "You take the genitourinary system, for example, and you concentrate on that. You study the anatomy of the kidneys and the physiology of the kidneys and all the things that can go wrong with them, and at the same time you see patients in the hospital with kidney and bladder disease—just as a student, of course—and at the same time you study your textbooks on the anatomy and physiology and pathology of the kidneys and urinary tract. Then when you wrap that up, you go on to the gastrointestinal system and do the same thing, and then the cardiovascular system, and the nervous system, and the pulmonary system, and you follow the same pattern right on through all four years. We were seeing real patients in hospital beds the second day I was here as a freshman. And after all, why not? That's what medicine is all about, when you get right down to it: treating sick patients."

"But you never actually dissected a cadaver," I said.

"Me? No. The surgical Fellows prepared model dissections of the different organ systems for us to study, but there's no point to a medical student's wasting his time personally digging through all that skin and fat and fascia just to get down to those structures." He glanced across at the girl. "Of course, Hazel here helps the surgeons with the dissections whenever she can—but that's her choice, because she's on the surgical track. I'm on the family-practice track myself."

"Track?"

"Right. Everybody selects a track—a route of study or a special interest," the girl explained. "It can be surgery, or internal medicine, or OB-GYN or family practice or whatever. It's sort of like picking a major in college. Everybody gets a lot of everything, but you get a whole lot more in the track you choose than in other things. And when you have elective time, you pick electives related to your track, too."

"But once you choose a track, you're stuck with it?"

"Oh, no, you can change tracks if you want to. Some do, too, but not too many."

"Do you actually spend any time at all in basic science laboratories?"

"A little, but not too much."

"What about lectures?"

"We have lots of lectures," Hazel said. "Good ones, too. Good lecturers. Nobody sits there and goes to sleep. In some of the really important lectures—pathology, for instance—we have a crazy feedback system so that the prof knows whether he's getting through or not, and the students can stop him if he's going over their heads. Up in the lecture amphitheater every student's seat has a panel of buttons. Any time the prof wants to during his lecture he can stop and ask people to rate how well they understood what he just said. Each student pushes a rating button by his seat, and the prof sees the result on a panel down at the lectern and he knows right then if it's gone right past everybody, or if almost everybody got it, or what. Same way, a student can push a 'hold it' button when something goes by that he didn't get, and when the prof sees lots of lights on his panel he knows he has to go back and try that particular item a different way. It's great for the after-lunch blahs, too. Keeps everybody on his toes."

"So what happens when you finish all four years of the medical school here? Do you just automatically move into a Fellowship at the Clinic?"

The girl laughed. "No way," she said. "That would be

dreamy, but it doesn't work that way. All the seniors enter the National Internship Matching Plan, just like senior medical students everywhere else in the country. They list hospitals where they'd like to go, in order of preference, and the hospitals list the students they'd like to have the most, in order of preference, and then the computer matches the lists, and on March 15 the students find out where they're going to go. Of course, Mayo can put some of their own graduates high on their list, if they want to, and often do, but they're looking for new blood from other places too."

The girl spread her hands. "Personally, if I'm still on the surgical track, I'd like to stay here if I can qualify, even though I might get to do more actual surgery sooner some other place. The staff surgeons and senior Fellows here do almost all the actual surgery, since it's a private practice and there aren't any charity patients to toss to the house doctors—but the quality of teaching here and the reputation of the place just can't be beat. If they'll let me stay here, I will."

"Not me," Larry said, "no way in the world. Their family practice training is brand new here, and for my money it stinks. They just don't know what they're doing. The truth is, they've got no *need* for family practitioners at Mayo. They only started the program because they saw the nationwide statistics on family practice, saw the big groundswell developing in family medicine and figured they'd have to toss it a bone if they wanted to recruit students for the medical school. But basically it's silly here. Mayo Clinic is a super-specialty oriented organization. They don't even know what a family practitioner *is*, except for this picture they have of some ignorant rube off in Central Nowhere who sends them his tough cases. So what they've set up for graduate training in family practice is really pretty sad. Maybe it'll get better when they get used to it, but it's going to take a long time."

I got a better idea of what Larry Silverman was talking about that afternoon when I rented a car and drove out to the tiny little town of Kasson, some fifteen miles west of Rochester, to pay a visit to—of all things—the Mayo Clinic. That's what it said on the wall of the handsome, new, sprawling one-story brick building that looked exactly like a newly built small-town doctor's office. It was lunch hour when I arrived, and the waiting room, shaded against the hot sun, was empty except for a nurse behind the reception counter. She escorted me back to an office-consulting room where Dr. Perrier was busy devouring a huge sandwich and drinking cocoa out of a thermos.

Annette Perrier was a striking woman of about thirty, an almost breathtakingly beautiful woman, instantly demolishing any lingering suspicions I might have had that today's women doctors all had mustaches and bad complexions. Petite and trim, she was dressed more casually than the Clinic doctors in Rochester—but dungarees and thin jersey blouses were clearly not *de rigueur* in her office. Brushing aside my apology for interrupting her lunch, she shoved the sandwich aside and led me out to show me her office. "I'm just a compulsive lunch-eater," she explained. "The truth is, I don't really *need* that sandwich. I know that. But every day I eat it, just the same."

The building had ample office space for three doctors, including consulting rooms, examining rooms, a very small X-ray room, and small minor surgery ("We also use it for revising casts and putting on splints and things like that"), a treatment room with electrocardiogram and a variety of other instruments, and the nurses' "shot room" where immunizations and medications were given, with a tiny autoclave in one corner. "I don't know why we have that," Dr. Perrier said, "since we hardly ever use it, but they had a room full of them in storage at the Clinic, so we got one. Mostly we use disposables out here—syringes, needles, everything. We use the X ray to check for sprains or fractures and to take chest X rays; anything much more complex goes into town."

Back in her office, the doctor explained their operation. "I'm a GP, a family practitioner, board certified by the American Academy of Family Physicians. I'm one of the first on the Mayo Clinic staff—this is really all very new to them—and one of the very few, too. Oh, yes, I'm a bona-fide staff doctor at the Clinic, salary and all the rest on the same basis as any of the rest of the staff, except that I'm sort of an ugly duckling." She laughed. "I mean, I can't actually *do* anything very much. This office is what they call an 'outreach facility,' the Clinic's way of reaching out to surrounding communities. It'll ultimately work into their graduate training program for family practitioners. This is just a wee little town, not even a thousand people, but there are lots of farm families in the area, and I take care of the routine family medical care, treat colds and diaper rash and earaches, prenatal care, all that sort of thing."

"But you take the women in to St. Mary's to deliver them, I assume."

She shook her head. "All the OB patients go to Rochester Methodist now—part of the 'division of labor' plan the hospitals are putting into effect. As for delivering the babies, up until a couple of years ago I *didn't* deliver them. When they were ready, I had to send them into the hospital in Rochester and a Clinic OB man delivered them. The Clinic didn't even want me to assist. I caught one by accident out here, now and then, but not very often." Dr. Perrier laughed. "Well, we had a big fat fight about *that* little setup, and I won. I had pretty good OB training in my residency and plenty of support in case of problems, and the patients didn't *want* somebody else delivering them—so now I take them in and deliver them myself."

"In other words, even a big place like Mayo Clinic can be whipped in a fight."

"Let's just say they can change." She sighed. "Unfortunately, there are still lots of things that I don't get to do here. I may find surgery that needs doing, but I don't get to do it. I may see accident cases, but this is just an outpost; all I'm supposed to do is keep the victims alive long enough to get them in to Rochester. If I run into a fracture much worse than a cracked rib, I don't handle it. It's really very restrictive, and I sometimes wonder if the Clinic truly knows what it's doing. They almost seem *afraid* of family practice—it's alien to their whole setup—but they seem to feel they've got to do *something* with it. So they have this place, and there's a larger, older facility up north in Zumbrota, and they're planning a couple of others. I don't know if it's going to work out or not. Of course, I have the greatest consultation in the world just a few miles away, and the patients come back and see me when they get back home, but by then the fun and games are all over. And there's no practical way I can follow them in Rochester. I'm not even supposed to *be* there—I'm supposed to be out here. True, I have plenty of time off, with family practice Fellows to relieve me, but all the same . . ." Her voice trailed off.

"You don't sound too happy," I said.

"It's not a completely happy situation," she said. "I'm like a fifth wheel—not truly very important to the Clinic and not all that important to the patients either. I serve a purpose, but it's not the vital, baseline medical purpose a family practitioner ought to be fulfilling in a community like this. I'm always in the shadow of that tall gray building."

"But you're here just the same," I said.

"Oh, yes. There's lots to learn and sick people to care for. There's a sort of a crazy medical challenge to it, too, walking into a setup that doesn't make the least bit of sense, a setup that shouldn't work at *all* and trying to *make* it work the best you can. I don't know what's going to happen, and I guess I'm kind of curious to find out."

"But you're not planning to spend your life at it," I said.

"My *life?*" She laughed. "No, I don't think so. Not like some of those guys on the staff, three generations deep into the Mayo Clinic. I'll work on it for a while, but then I think I'll probably move on."

Later that same Friday, in the cool of evening, Roger Barton was driving his car south on Highway 90 to the Iowa border and on toward home in Mason City. The evening was beautiful, the sky still luminous. As he drove down through the gently rolling farm country he reached an area where an early hay crop had just been mowed on either side of the highway. Roger tipped his head back and inhaled deeply. To his utter amazement, he discovered he could actually *smell* that new-mown hay, unlike any other smell in the world, thick and rich and fragrant.

It hit him with such impact that his eyes filled with tears and he almost had to pull off the road. *My God,* he thought, *how long has it been since I smelled that smell? Not since I was a little kid, not once in the last thirty years—and I've lived in Iowa all my life.*

Earlier in the afternoon Roger had had his final meeting with Dr. DeVore in his office in the Mayo Building. Roger had displayed a large green envelope filled with pills. "I decided to go along with Dr. Fried's little research game," he said. "After all, I figure, what have I got to lose? There was sure nothing helping my nose when I came here. You ordered those other pills, but he said it wouldn't hurt to take his too. I started them first thing this morning. But I can't say I notice any difference."

"They may just be the sugar pills anyway," Dr. DeVore said. "Nobody will know for sure until the study is over. But as far as your asthma is concerned, as well as your plugged-up nose, I think you're going to get a great deal of help from the medicine I ordered, regardless of Dr. Fried's pills— especially now that we have a clear handle on what some of your allergic triggers are. Let's go along exactly the way we discussed, with you taking the medicines—actually *taking* them—and also carefully avoiding the trigger allergens we found on the skin tests. I'd like to check you again in a month to see how you're doing. If nothing much is happening, then we can go on to desensitization."

The doctor pulled Roger's chart forward on the desk. "Now let's talk about these other things," he said. Carefully, step by step, he reviewed the results of the many studies Roger had had during the week, explaining why they had been done, what the results were and what they meant. "Chest X ray clear—cardiogram normal, blood sugar normal, these blood chemistries measuring kidney and liver function all normal, these general metabolic screening tests we like to do also normal. Your blood lipids—cholesterol and triglycerides—are well above the normal range, and the distribution—the ratio of high density lipids—is not very encouraging." He looked up at Roger. "This pattern is certainly partly due to the less than prudent diet you've been indulging in. You did have a session with our dietitian this morning? Fine. They may also be due in part to your obesity, or to genetic factors, or your cigarette smoking, or some combination of all of those things. But all of these factors except your genetic makeup are controllable and reversible. We've already talked about what you can do about all this if you choose to. You either will or you won't, but we'll go all over it with you again in a month or so when I check out these other things."

"Well, maybe I'll do something," Roger said gloomily.

"Why not?" DeVore said. "You've impressed me from the first as a sensible young man who might want to dig in and get your health under control. As it is right now, you've got a chance to reverse things, slow them down, if you can just get hold of the reins. If you don't, you're about ninety-five percent certain to have serious coronary heart disease about ten years from now, and then it's going to be too late to change a lot. So why not get hold of the reins right now?"

Dr. DeVore went back to the chart. "Your twenty-four-hour urine test, the one with the big jug, came out all right, and so did the twenty-four-hour sputum. The breathing tests—well, you still have pretty surprising capacity, considering the asthma and the chronic bronchitis and the smoking, but it's certainly not what it ought to be. You've already got real chronic bronchial obstructive disease, still reversible, but very much there. You don't need *me* to tell you about the risk of smoking—you know that as well as I do—but if you really need to have a doctor tell you point-blank, 'Stop smoking, Roger,' then I'm telling you. Just bite the bullet and stop and don't start again. And like they say in the TV business, do it *now*."

The doctor pushed back in his seat and looked at Roger. "Okay, that covers those things—but we still haven't touched on the one really immediate and dangerous threat, have we?"

Roger shifted uncomfortably. "You mean the high blood pressure?"

Dr. DeVore nodded.

"Some help you are," Roger said bitterly. "I come up here to get my allergies fixed and you give me high blood pressure."

DeVore grinned. "I don't suppose you're thanking me much for finding it. But it's there, all the same."

"I still think it's just that Mickey Mouse machine you've got up on East Sixteen," Roger said.

"I don't think even *you* believe that."

"Well, I'm just going to have to get another blood-pressure cuff," Roger said.

"Fine," Dr. DeVore said dryly. "Just get one that works, this time. Meanwhile, I understand you had a long go-around with Dr. Parker over in the hypertensive disease section yesterday and that he has a schedule of medications set up for you to start on, as well as the diet program. But just to be sure you understand it, I want to review it again right now, if you've got a little time."

I had dinner with Roger Barton that evening in the Elizabethan Room of the Kahler Hotel before he checked out to start on his journey home. I'd run into him a dozen times during the week past as we went our various ways, and we had struck up an acquaintance. Now he greeted me in the Mayo Building lobby like a long-lost brother and nothing would do but he take me to dinner. "It's not too bad a place to eat," he said. "Even pretty good, sometimes, though the service leaves a lot to be desired and the wine cellar—" he shook his head— "simply awful."

We took an out-of-the-way table and over a double Jack Daniels with a dash of Southern Comfort in it he began talking quite freely about his experience at the Mayo Clinic. I listened, nodding and making appropriate sounds at appropriate points. During my visits to Rochester I had chatted informally with literally dozens of patients in waiting rooms, out in the entry halls of the Mayo Building, or in the hotel lobbies or elevators, but few were quite as open and unguarded as Roger Barton seemed this evening. Clearly, here was a young man who was certain beyond doubt that his own experiences and opinions were the most fascinating topics of conversation in the world.

"So how do you add it up, now that you've finished here?" I asked him finally. "How do these Mayo people stack up to other doctors you've seen before?"

"Well, I've never really been desperately ill," Roger said, suddenly sober. "I mean, no cancer, no heart attacks, no sudden frightful need for surgery, so I can't really say on that account. But I can tell you this: I've been seeing doctors all my life, and I've never had a medical experience like this one before. I've never had an exam so totally thorough, with doctors so obviously determined to leave no stone unturned. Of course, you could live without some of the irritations—the long waits to see doctors, the awkward last-minute changes of plans, a few really irritating people to put up with—but where are you going to escape that? And they're pretty damned peremptory, too. When you come here, as far as they're concerned, your time is one hundred percent theirs. They don't give a damn *what* else you might want to do. They parcel your time out as if they owned it and say, 'You be *here* at such and such a time' and you by God had better be there or you've lost a day. And then when you get there they let you sit for six hours. I think with better planning they could have wrapped up my exam in three and a half days instead of five—well, maybe not; that would have taken awfully tight planning—but really, all this is insignificant compared to what really matters."

He flagged a passing waiter to come replace a water glass that he fancied had a bit of lipstick on its rim. "What's significant, to me, is the incredible thoroughness of the exam, the *determination* to be thorough, no matter what else. That's first. Second is the feeling you get that these people are after *results* for their patients. There's none of this business of, 'Well, well, that's a rare and interesting disease you have, my good man, but there's nothing to be done about it. Come back in two years and let us see how bad it's gotten.' These people are real hawks for doing something. They didn't build this place on vague promises. They built it on taking sick people and making them well, or at least making them feel better, or at the *very* least making them *think* something has been done for them. They're clever and slick, and they've got a lot to offer, and if they possibly can they're going to see to it that the patient is better off when he walks out of here than he was when he walked in."

Roger laughed. "Some of it's kind of silly, in a way," he said. "I mentioned the blood pressure and the overweight and how steamed up they seemed to be about this, didn't I? Well, I spent an hour this morning, one solid hour, with a dietitian, and she took that time going over a diet with me to help me cut down my salt intake, cut down my cholesterol level and knock off three pounds of weight a month, all at one whack. Well, hell! That woman was straight out of Fairyland. I listened to her and watched her work out her little chart of foods, and I could hardly believe my eyes. I could no more stay on that diet for three days than I could fly to Turkey by flapping my arms. Hell, I doubt if I could even gag it down. Ninety milligrams of salt a day." He sprinkled a small dash of salt from the table shaker into his palm and tossed it into his mouth. "That's ninety milligrams of salt right there, and I don't even have my steak yet. I'm a salt-eater, I always have been and I told her so, too, and she smiled and nodded and wrote down ninety milligrams of salt. No fried foods. No fat on the meat. Three eggs a *week*. Four ounces of beef is *dinner*. No butter. Two fresh vegetables for lunch and two fresh vegetables for dinner. Yuck."

"So what did you tell her?" I asked.

"Tell her? What could I tell her? She was doing her job the best she knew how, and she couldn't do any other job under the circumstances, so what was there to tell her? She finished up filling in the diet booklet and put my name on it and handed it to me and I thanked her and she went along her way to see the next patient. And who knows, maybe I can use that booklet somehow as some kind of a guide to modify what I eat—but as a diet? Insane."

Roger ordered another double bourbon and went on. "Fortunately, some of their other recommendations made a whole lot more sense. I'm going to have to do some thinking. I have a hunch this DeVore chap is going to keep goading me until I do. And that's the third remarkable thing that hits me about this place, maybe the most important thing of all. This Clinic is huge, and it's got to be impersonal. You'd think it would have to be about as impersonal and uncaring as any medical institution could possibly get, and yet guys like Dr. DeVore seem to have this weird, incredible knack for making you feel that they *really give* a damn about you as a human being. I don't know what it is, exactly, but it *can't* be phony—it's got to be real. Partly it's the time they spend. I had to wait, a couple of times, but there wasn't a doctor I saw here who seemed to be in any big hurry once he got around to seeing me. They didn't *waste* time, but every one of them took the time that was necessary."

The steaks arrived at last, and we settled down to a delicious dinner. "Another part of it," Roger continued between bites, "is just their overall approach to patients. With ninety percent of the doctors you see nowadays, you're in and out of their offices so fast you don't know what hit you. They listen to your chest, ask you half a dozen rapid-fire questions and then sit writing out prescriptions while you're still answering. They don't care whether those prescriptions do any good or not. What they care about is the fifty additional patients they've still got to crank through their offices that day, and until they get rid of you they can't get the next one in. Well, these Mayo docs didn't do that. The prescriptions they wrote for me had some thought behind them, some real rationale, and they cared enough to let me know what to watch out for and what to do in case something went wrong."

Roger sighed and helped himself to the wine. "Of course, what matters most from my viewpoint is clearing up a lifelong problem. Well, it may sound silly, but for the first time in years I honestly think I may have a chance to *beat* this asthma and this nasal allergy and that somebody up here is willing to hang tough with me until I do. And to top it all off, the price isn't all that high, not for what you get. This is all private practice, you know. This is the kind of medical care that's supposed to be so godawful costly that nobody but millionaires can afford it—at least that's what Senator Kennedy keeps telling us. This is the kind of medical care that's supposed to be so prohibitively costly that it breaks people's backs and reduces families to financial ruin. Far too costly to tolerate in our society and all that slop. Well, do you know what's *really* too costly to tolerate in our society? *Automobiles,* that's what. Not private medical care. You know what my bill was at the Mayo Clinic for this week-long workup? Seven hundred twenty-three dollars and forty-three cents— that's how much. Well, I'm no millionaire, and I don't like to pay doctors any more than anybody else, but that bill doesn't look so intolerable to me, considering what I got for it. About what you'd pay for a real wreck of a used car."

"People have to have their cars," I said.

Roger shook his head in disgust. "People have to have their health, too," he said. "I got something of lasting value for my seven hundred and twenty-three dollars, maybe something of value to my *life.* Well, I've got a buddy that sells cars down in Mason City. I know how many people there are on mechanics' salaries or farm-hand salaries or mill workers' salaries who think *nothing* of paying six thousand dollars every three years for cars that are so badly built they fall apart on the road in two years. I know how many people pay five hundred a month *rent* for an ordinary apartment in some new complex, and I know how many are spending eight to twenty grand each for these campers and mobile homes that are crowding us off the highways—and they're nothing but *vacation toys.* And then the federal government tries to tell me that private medical care is too costly for us to tolerate in our society! Well, maybe I'll feel different about my Clinic bill six months from now when nothing has happened and it all looks like money down the drain, but somehow I doubt it. Say, you know something?" He looked up suddenly. "They must have gotten a new chef around here. This steak tastes absolutely great! And it smells even better."

When Dr. Jerry Whitehead made his rounds that evening at Rochester Methodist Hospital with his retinue of Fellows, medical students and nurses trailing behind, Millie Hulbert was waiting like a panther to pounce on him. "I want to go home," she told him.

"I was afraid you were going to say that." Dr. Whitehead reviewed her chart, inspected her dressings, examined her arm on the incision side for any signs of edema, then listened to her heart and lungs. "Temp?" he asked the nurse.

"One-o-one point two this afternoon."

"That's what I thought," Whitehead said. "She has some rales in the right lung base, too, that weren't there this morning." He looked critically at Millie. "What do you mean by 'home'? Back to Denver?"

"Well, Tim MacMichael invited Ada and me to come up to the lake for a couple of days. Then I thought I might fly home next Tuesday."

The surgeon shook his head, slowly but firmly. "Mrs. Hulbert, you're crowding it," he told her. "It's just too soon, even on general principles, and on top of that you're spiking a post-op fever and may be developing a little pneumonitis in the right side of your chest there. I'm not going to let you budge for at least two more days, if then. And don't ask Tim, either. He won't make me change my mind."

The woman looked disappointed, but Whitehead knew she'd go along. The previous evening he had spent most of an hour talking with Millie Hulbert about the findings at surgery and the treatment options available, and she had agreed wholeheartedly with his recommendation not to pursue further treatment at this time.

In the course of their talks Millie had found herself liking Jerry Whitehead more and more. She didn't know what it was, except that somewhere along the line she began sensing that the man really cared about what was best for her, acting more like a sensitive human being than the surgical automaton he had seemed when she first saw him. "I've seen some of the women who've had the X-ray or chemotherapy treatments," she'd said, "and some of them were just miserable. Maybe if I were a younger woman I'd say, 'let's do it,' but at my age—I don't think so. I'm just too old to want to be heroic. And, maybe the surgery really did get it all."

Now the surgeon said, "You check with Tim and let him

know that you're grounded for a while longer. But meantime, we need to plan. Further treatment or no further treatment, you're going to need follow-up. You should have a thorough going-over at six months and again in a year."

"I suppose I could come back here," Millie said dubiously.

"At one year, that would be good. Maybe you could visit your friends out here next summer. But at six months it shouldn't be necessary. Do you know any surgeons in Denver?"

She laughed. "There's the nice young man who took care of that melanoma—but I don't think he knows very much."

"Maybe he knows more than you think," Whitehead said. "But if you'd rather, I can give you the name of a woman in Denver you could see sometime right after New Year's. Dr. Chris Moscowitz. She's a very good surgeon and an old friend of mine." Dr. Whitehead printed the name and address on the back of one of his own cards and handed it to Millie. "If you'd like, I'll send her a résumé of what we've done and found and planned so she'll be up to date. Then next June I'd like to see you here, if you can work it. Meanwhile, let's concentrate on clearing up your chest and getting rid of your fever so we can spring you out of here."

He shook her hand then and moved along with his entourage. Millie Hulbert went back to the letter she was writing, finished it and sealed it—a letter to a son containing as little information as possible about her condition and a great deal about her plans: back to Denver as soon as she could manage, then divide Thanksgiving and Christmas between the kids and then maybe a trip down to San Diego to visit Muriel during the really cold months—yes, that would be nice; Denver *did* get cold in winter. She put away her writing materials, shifted to try to get comfortable in the hospital bed, examined it critically for the fortieth time—*nasty hard thing, and they insist upon rolling up the end as if I were an old fossil with heart failure*—then took off her glasses and rubbed her eyes. She ran through the television stations in thirty seconds flat, snorted and turned the machine off again. For another ten minutes she fidgeted, sneaking looks at the telephone. *Two more days here because of a little fever*, she thought. *As if I were some sort of delicate flower. Well, nonsense. I'll just give Tim a call and see if he can't do something—*

She didn't, of course. She struggled with the idea, remembered what Dr. Whitehead had said, suspected he wasn't joking and finally went back to reading a dull book. "No wonder hospital bills are so high," she grumbled, "with people kept in two days longer than they have any need to be. But then—" she pursed her lips in disapproval—"I suppose there's always Medicare."

11

Rochester, Minnesota / 1910–1939

The decades of the 1910s and 1920s marked the heyday of Charles Horace and William James Mayo as world-famous surgeons and the flowering of the Mayo Clinic as a major American medical institution.

The practice in Rochester, and especially the surgical practice, had grown almost beyond belief; the streets of Rochester were crowded with the horse carts and buggies and wagons of patients and then, more and more, with automobiles. The Mayo brothers and Starr Judd were working constantly in their surgeries, and more staff doctors were taken on constantly to support their work. Physicians well trained in internal medicine were brought in to see the growing numbers of nonsurgical patients the Clinic had attracted. More hotels were built to handle the influx of people.

This was the period when the Mayo brothers began to make their mark in the national surgical establishment not as a couple of rubes working out in a corn patch somewhere but as a couple of surgeons to be seriously reckoned with.

In a way those other surgeons could hardly be blamed, at first, for being skeptical of the claims these young men were making. They simply couldn't comprehend the sheer volume of surgery that was being done in this small Minnesota town. As a typical example of their consternation, a world-renowned surgeon from Boston would take the podium at a surgical conference in the East and deliver a lengthy and erudite paper on surgical removal of the gall bladder based on nine such cases he had performed in the course of the previous year. When the time for discussion came, a young man named W. J. Mayo would stand up in the back of the room and take sharp issue with the surgical technique the noted surgeon had just described. One could get far better results, Mayo proclaimed, if one did the procedure like *this* instead of like *that*. "Ahem, very interesting comment," the noted surgeon would say. "But tell me, Doctor, on what experience are you basing your criticism?"

And the young man would say, in his flat Midwest twang, "Well, Doctor, my brother, Charlie, and I have done one hundred and twenty-three of these procedures in the last nine months, and we've gotten lots better results than most reports we've read about."

One hundred and twenty-three gall bladders. *One hundred and twenty-three?* Good God! Were they taking out every gall bladder in Minnesota? Or was this young man just a fraud?

Such disbelief was a problem for Will and Charlie for a while. People simply would not believe them. They would submit a paper reviewing their results in a series of ninety-six gastrectomies for publication in a major surgical journal and the editor would reject it as pure chicanery; many fine surgeons had not done more than four or five gastrectomies in their careers, and here these Mayo brothers were claiming to have done almost 100! Presently, however, a few surgeons with impeccable credentials and high reputations decided to put an end to these extravagant claims once and for all. They would go out to Rochester themselves and see just what *was* going on.

They came back home with their jaws sagging. One such man was Dr. Carl Beck of Chicago, whose surgery Charles Mayo had visited on one of his "brain picking" trips. Dr. Beck had been startled to hear that this stocky young fellow from Rochester now claimed to know a great deal about gall-bladder surgery. In fact, he was amazed that the man should even have attempted the operation. At the urging of Dr. Nicholas Senn, another surgeon astonished at some cases that Will Mayo had recently reported at an American Medical Association meeting, Beck got on the train for Rochester. The following day he observed both brothers doing surgery with uncommon craft and skill. He toured St. Mary's Hospital, met the Mayos' partners and visited their offices. Among other things, he saw the hordes of patients thronging the waiting rooms, the carriages tied up to every available hitching post and other signs of a practice enormous enough to keep a great city medical center busy.

By the end of his visit, any question Dr. Beck had about the work the Mayos were doing was completely dispelled. These men were not exaggerating. If anything they were *understating* their surgical experience. What was more, a surgeon could learn a great deal from these two men, and Beck decided then and there to come back to visit them often. Nor was he the only one to learn something from this experience. The Mayo brothers learned, too. From then on whenever their word was questioned by anyone, they had a single answer: "Come to Rochester and see."

More and more surgeons began doing just that. Some merely came to snoop, to satisfy their curiosity or make sure the Mayos were not charlatans. But many returned to Rochester again and again. Visitors were welcome to observe any operation that was being done, whether it were simple or difficult and whether it went well or badly. And there seemed to be no shortage of things for them to observe and learn in the Mayos' surgeries. Between them, in the early 1900s, the two brothers were doing 4,000 operations a year. It was not uncommon for Will Mayo to do eight to ten operations in a single day. In the twelve years ending with 1902 the brothers had completed a total of 500 gall-bladder operations; they did the second 500 in the following eighteen months. In 1905 Dr. Will delivered a discussion on 500 cases of gastric surgery that he had done. And Charlie was beginning to gather a respectable series of thyroidectomies.

Surgical failures? They had them and did not try to hide them. On the contrary, they would often report them and try to analyze why those particular cases had been failures. What was more, they did not go along with surgeons who insisted that as long as the patient was still breathing when he was wheeled out of the operating room, the surgery was successful, even if he might die ten minutes later. To them any patient who died during his postoperative recovery period was a surgical death as far as they were concerned.

Such candor did much to enhance the brothers' reputation, and the trickle of visiting surgeons became a steadily expanding stream. No longer were other surgeons questioning the Mayos' claims; instead they were inviting Will and Charlie to present papers at major surgical meetings. Famous surgeons in the great cities were beginning to acknowledge publicly the skills these brothers were demonstrating and the surgical advancements they were pioneering. Probably it was Dr. Will's bold innovations in performing gastrectomies—removing a portion of the stomach in the treatment of peptic ulcer disease, gastric cancer or gastric obstruction—that brought him his greatest fame and recognition in the early 1900s.

Interestingly enough, these visiting surgeons who came to observe the Mayos at work were also responsible, to a large extent, for extending the reach of the Mayos' practice far beyond the Midwest. These men went home to their own practices—but when faced with cases beyond their own capabilities they would refer their patients to the Mayo brothers. As a result, the Mayos more and more were seeing patients who had come to them from one side of the continent to the other.

Meanwhile, other aspects of Mayo Clinic work began growing to catch up with the surgery. Until a regular staff of interns began coming to St. Mary's Hospital, anesthesia in the operating room was given by nurses, most particularly by Miss Alice Magaw. Miss Magaw became a veritable expert at the administration of ether anesthesia (she soon discarded chloroform as far too dangerous, even while practically every surgeon in the country was still using it). She found new ways to administer the ether on a gauze screen over the patient's face with a generous supply of oxygen to minimize the risk of ether pneumonia or overdosage. She also recognized the importance of a quiet and gentle approach to the frightened patient and learned a multitude of ways to determine when sufficient anesthesia had been given in order to avoid disasters. In 1904 Miss Magaw was invited to address a meeting of the Minnesota State Medical Society to report on her experience with 11,000 anesthesias, and soon anesthetists from all over the country were traveling to Rochester to observe the work of the Mayo brothers' unsurpassed nurse-anesthetist first hand.

Other physicians joined the Clinic group in steady succession. In 1905 a full-time pathologist, Dr. Louis B. Wilson, joined the Rochester group. One of his early contributions was a technique for fastening a bit of tissue taken from a patient still on the operating table between a couple of pieces of punky wood, setting the whole unit outside the window to freeze in the raw January air, and then slicing off thin sections with a razor blade. With a fast stain applied to the thin-sliced tissue, he could examine the cells under the microscope and tell the surgeon if cancer was present, then and there. Bit by bit Wilson refined this crude "frozen section" technique, using compressed carbon dioxide to freeze the tissue and a microtome blade to cut the slices of tissue extremely thin. Within a few months he had the technique down so well that he could give the surgeon a report on a specimen within two to five minutes while the patient was still asleep on the operating table—the basic technique of frozen sections that is still used in every major operating room in the country today.

Presently yet another pathologist joined the group. But something new also began to happen: One by one, physicians who had no interest at all in surgery began joining the group to serve as general diagnosticians and medical specialists for the many Clinic patients suffering from medical rather than surgical illnesses. In addition, for the first time, doctors came to Mayo's to do nothing but research work.

In the case of young Dr. Henry Plummer, the Mayo brothers struck pure gold. Perhaps no other single partner ultimately proved of greater lasting value to the group. Plummer was a strange man with the markings of genius about him; his influence and impact on the early Clinic were profound. Without this quiet genius in those early days there might be no Mayo Clinic as we know it today.

Young Dr. Plummer was practicing with his father in a small town north of Rochester when Will Mayo encountered him, almost by accident, and was deeply impressed by the young man's broad knowledge of hematology—the medical field dealing with the diagnosis and treatment of blood diseases. Since so much of hematology involves clinical laboratory work, Mayo hired Plummer primarily to set up and organize clinical laboratory facilities for the Clinic. This Plummer did—but it soon became clear that nobody was going to tuck him away in a pigeonhole as a "laboratory man." He was a skilled diagnostician both for surgical and medical illnesses and was soon making himself indispensable as a clinical consultant to every other doctor in the group—so much so that he was soon accepted as a full partner in the growing nucleus of the Mayo Clinic staff.

One area that particularly intrigued Plummer was the study of thyroid disease and the function of the thyroid gland, a field of medicine in which very little was known at the time. It was also an extremely confusing field of study, involving a group of illnesses which seemed impossible to diagnose correctly and equally impossible to treat. True, surgery to remove goiters or tumors of the thyroid gland was being done at the time, and in fact Charlie Mayo was establishing this as one of his surgical specialties. Yet an alarming number of such surgical patients would become violently ill following their surgery for totally obscure reasons and would often even die for no apparent reason at all and despite everything the surgeon could do.

Henry Plummer set about studying the behavior of the thyroid gland in exquisite detail, both in the laboratory and in the thyroid patients who came to the Clinic as well. Presently, at a time when no one knew anything to speak of about thyroid hormone or how it worked, Plummer was able to distinguish two or more quite different kinds of surgical thyroid disease and, by minute observation of the patients, pinpoint in advance which ones would be likely to suffer these violent "thyroid storms" following surgery and which would not. He also developed procedures that would largely prevent this sort of postsurgical disaster from happening. In this work he and Charlie Mayo worked hand in hand, and it was this partnership of acute diagnosis, clinical research and skillful surgery that resulted for the first time in making necessary thyroid surgery plausible and reasonably safe as a surgical procedure. Later, Charlie and Henry Plummer were instrumental in bringing Dr. Edward C. Kendall, a young biochemist from New York, to Rochester to try to refine an extract of thyroid gland he had prepared from slaughterhouse thyroid glands. Ultimately, early in 1915, Kendall finally isolated a small amount of an active hormone from the thyroid—a substance he called thyroxin.

But Henry Plummer was far more than just a physician. He was a true Renaissance man, an idea man, a tinkerer and inventor and thinker and designer. When the time came that a new building had to be constructed to house the Mayo Clinic offices, laboratories and X-ray facilities, Plummer was the one who took a long look at the growing and varied needs of the group and then set down a detailed building design to fulfill those needs. When the Mayo brothers and the other physicians found the patient load so heavy that they were wasting enormous amounts of time during office hours in the Clinic just getting patients into examining rooms for the doctors to see them, Plummer devised an ingenious signal system of colored flags outside each examining door, much like railroad semaphores, with one color assigned to each doctor and the position of the flag indicating if a patient in a room was waiting to be seen, or the doctor was with the patient then, or the doctor had finished and the room was empty. With this system the nurses could tell at a glance which doctor was where, which doctor was free, which room was free, and so forth. This system of colored signals worked so well that, with very minor modification (colored lights instead of flags), it is still used today in the modern Mayo Clinic.

Another enduring contribution of Dr. Plummer had to do with patient records. When the practice was small, it had made sense to keep medical charts in large manila folders in file drawers. But the growing Mayo Clinic soon ran into trouble with chart-handling. Plummer tackled the problem and came up with a supremely reasonable scheme. He designed a new, uniform patient chart, small in size, to be prepared for each new patient. The first such chart under the new system, for Patient #1, was opened on July 19, 1907. Ever since then each new Clinic patient has had a similar chart, numbered in sequence, and once a patient has a number assigned, that individual number remains his forever.

The other part of Plummer's chart-handling system was particularly ingenious. He devised a pneumatic tube system, with capsules just big enough to accommodate the new charts, and then simply ran the pneumatic tubes to deliver the charts wherever they might be needed. It worked splendidly then, and it still works splendidly today with practically no modification.

Plummer was not an easy man to have around. He was stubborn, often preoccupied to the point of absent-mindedness and had a way of coming up with bright ideas at two o'clock in the morning and then stirring somebody up to sit and argue them out with him until dawn. But there was probably no other single man besides the Mayo brothers themselves who left a more permanent mark on the growth and operation of the Mayo Clinic. When yet a bigger Clinic building was needed in 1923, Plummer again did the designing. It was so soundly built that it is still a landmark in Rochester today and an essential, still-operating part of the Mayo complex—now appropriately known as the Plummer Building.

Other changes came to the Clinic during the crucial years between 1905 and 1915. In 1907 Mrs. Maude H. Mellish was hired to serve as librarian to the rapidly growing institution. In addition, she began an even more specialized service: assisting Mayo doctors in writing medical papers for publication—actually providing an editorial service for them. As a result, doctors around the country were amazed at the way Mayo papers always seemed so excellently written, so lucid and to the point. This work proved so useful that today a large Editorial Department exists at the modern Mayo to ensure that scientific publications emanating from the staff doctors and others are uniformly well presented.

At about the same time it became clear that something had to be done to maintain coherent business records for the Clinic. In 1908 the Mayos hired Harry J. Harwick, a twenty-one-year-old bank teller from Winona, Minnesota, to help with the problem. Harwick soon arranged a new, sensible system for keeping patient accounts and in 1910 became purchasing agent for the entire group. Ultimately Harwick was appointed the Mayo Clinic's overall business manager, a position he fulfilled until his retirement. At that time the job was taken over by his son, who had been well prepared for the position. In the summer of 1978 the elder Mr. Harwick died. A memorial service was held for him in the main-floor lobby of the Mayo Building, and the place was packed with people, including many doctors, patients and employees from the old days of the Clinic, come from the far corners to pay their final respects to this Mayo pioneer; his eulogy was read by Supreme Court Justice Harry Blackmun.

(By sheerest chance, while preparing this book, I encountered a granddaughter of the original Harry J. Harwick, now married and living on the East Coast. She had been born and raised in Rochester and spent many days in her grandfather's old house on 9th Avenue and 8th Street, S.W. "I remember the summers in that big old place," she said. "It was a huge house and had bay windows on all sides. When the weather got really hot in summer they would pull heavy curtains over those windows during the day to keep the heat out, the way they still do in the Middle West, so the whole house was dim and dark. But when I was a little girl I would crawl back of those curtains with a book and sit in the lighted bay windows to read." The old Harwick house still stands in Rochester, well-kept and handsome red brick with yellow trim. The bay windows are gone now, replaced with more modern windows, but when I walked by on a hot summer day I could see that the heavy curtains still were pulled.)

It was during these formative years of the Clinic that the Mayo brothers also suffered a major loss. During the later

1890s old Dr. Mayo, by then largely inactive in the practice, became increasingly irascible and difficult to have around, impatient in his demands and getting on everybody's nerves, including his own. Presently he began indulging his old wanderlust again, traveling far and wide for extended periods—even though he was well past eighty years old. His mind, however, was sharp as ever, and he sent back written reports from Florida, Cuba, Mexico, Canada, even an extensive five-month steamboat cruise to China and Japan upon which he embarked at the age of eighty-seven, enjoying his eighty-eighth birthday on board ship.

Back in Rochester following that sojourn, the elder Dr. Mayo devoted his efforts to a means of extracting alcohol from animal and vegetable wastes. One day the old man severely crushed his hand and part of his forearm in a machine that he was using and ultimately lost the limb to amputation. He never recovered from the blow to his general health and died shortly before his ninety-second birthday on March 6, 1911. Some months after his funeral a memorial association in Rochester raised funds for a monument to the pioneer physician. In good time a bronze statue was erected in a small but lovely Memorial Park, depicting the old doctor in the middle of a speech to a civic group, glasses in one hand, sheaf of disregarded notes in the other. It still stands there today. Mrs. Mayo died a few years later, in July 1915.

Until around 1914 virtually all the administration of the fast-growing Clinic and its many-sided medical activities had remained almost totally in the hands of the Mayo brothers themselves, without benefit of much coherent planning at all. If something sounded good for the practice, they consulted between themselves, made a decision, and it was done. But presently a point was reached that Will and Charlie themselves, with the constant pressure of their surgery, could no longer tend to all the administrative problems, even with Harry Harwick handling the business headaches and men like Henry Plummer providing both solid medical consultation and a fountain of ideas as well.

In fact, it was becoming clear that the organization could

no longer be managed as the Mayo Brothers' Clinic, operated and run for them alone as the chief constituents with the assistance of others. The time had come to move one step further and organize the Clinic as a complete, cooperative group practice of medicine, providing all the diagnostic and treatment facilities any patient might require, essentially housed under one roof and independent of any hospital or any public support. In this respect, it was totally unique. There were certainly groups of doctors who were already cooperating with each other, to some degree or another, at certain large county or university hospitals—but these Mayo Clinic men were private practitioners working in close cooperation with each other seeing private patients. They were, in short, a *private* group practice.

As such, absolute control finally passed out of the Mayo brothers' hands. Instead, a board of governors was appointed, including Dr. Plummer, Harry Harwick and a couple of younger members of the group as well as the two Mayo brothers. The rule of this board, however, was not heavy-handed, because a group of standing committees was also set up with virtually every member of the staff serving on one committee or another. In the long run it was those committees that determined what was needed, set policies, decided on activities of staff members and set the direction the Clinic should follow. The committees then took their decisions back to the board of governors, who were more likely to rubber-stamp them than debate them.

Indeed, many doctors in the group found themselves baffled at the *lack* of guidance and direction. They might take a bright idea to the board of governors, for example, and be told to present it to a committee, and then to a second committee, and then to yet a third, until it seemed there was no way to get anything done at all. Some of the men chafed at this procedure—but in the long run it had an odd way of working. If the idea was bad to start with, it would eventually wear itself out for sheer lack of action. On the other hand, if it had good qualities, somebody along the line would sit up and support it. The bugs would be hammered out, possible problems resolved and the final idea put into action—by which time it had often evolved from a merely good idea to an excellent one.

These years approaching the time of World War I were obviously vigorous growth years for the Mayo Clinic. They were also years in which worldwide fame and a long succession of medical honors came to the Mayo brothers, culminating in Will Mayo's induction as president of the American Medical Association in 1906 and Charlie's later succession to the same honored post in 1917.

All was not sweetness and light during this period, however. If the Mayos and their growing organization enjoyed the friendship and admiration of many of the leading surgeons in the country who recognized the quality of the work they were doing, they also fell victim to the vigorous dislike, even hatred, of many others who carried on a continuing and relentless campaign of spite against them. After all, the Mayo group had become conspicuously and spectacularly successful, well-to-do and world-famous—and there was nothing some doctors hated more than to see other doctors become successful, prosperous and famous when they were not. Multitudes of scruffy stories began circulating among doctors about the Mayos and their practice. They were not really great surgeons at all, it was said. They were just very ordinary surgeons with a knack for calling attention to themselves at every turn. They built those fantastic lists of cases they were constantly reporting by running a veritable cattle yard for patients in Rochester. They were not interested in the welfare of their patients, it was claimed, but only in doing spectacular and dangerous operations, and in order to do that, it was said, they would discount their fees for certain kinds of cases, pay the patients' train fare to Rochester and then bully them into accepting surgery whether there was any need for it or not.

Meanwhile, the stories said, the Mayos and their group were growing fantastically rich milking the patients' pocketbooks dry. This highly touted "private group practice" of theirs was really nothing more than a fancy fee-splitting ring, with patients handed from doctor to doctor so that everybody got a fee, and the Mayos themselves nothing more than glorified surgical profiteers.

The fact that such stories were demonstrably false did not in any way stop them from spreading, nor was there any effective way the Mayos could fight back. In a way, of course, it's easy to see why other physicians might be angry. It was bitter medicine for a doctor to have a patient he was treating hop onto a train for Rochester the moment there was any suggestion that he might need surgery. "Just going by the Mayos," the patient would say. And it was bitter business when a surgeon from St. Paul on a tour of the surgical clinics in Europe found himself asked: "St. Paul, Minnesota? Is that anywhere near Rochester?" Undoubtedly there were real grievances—but the rancor behind many of these anti-Mayo stories far transcended any real grievances.

Things weren't helped in the least by the way the public press caught on to the very real growing fame of the Mayo group and ballyhooed it to high heaven. If there is anything worse for a doctor's professional reputation than a succession of scurrilous underground stories, it is too much favorable attention from the public newspapers and major magazines—and here the Mayos *did* try to fight back. On one occasion, for example, a couple of lengthy and excessively adulatory articles about the Mayos and their career were written by lay reporters and published in mass-circulation national magazines. These articles were a terrible professional embarrassment to the Mayos. One in particular was so totally oblivious to the actual facts and published such grotesquely favorable exaggerations of the Mayos' surgical achievements that the brothers actually considered suing the author and the magazine and demanding retractions.

If the Mayos were distressed by this, their enemies were maliciously gleeful. Here was proof positive that these men in Rochester were irresponsible quacks, they said. They had obviously *commissioned* the article, deliberately breaking the most rigid taboo in the entire profession of medicine—the rule against self-advertising. Ultimately the brothers did the best thing they could think of: They wrote a public denial of responsibility for the article and a lengthy defense of their position and had it published in the *Journal of the American Medical Association*. They were undoubtedly angry and bitter; they felt they had always played the game by the rules, never in their lives knowingly seeking publicity other than reporting their work through the normal and completely acceptable channels in the professional meetings and journals. Experiences such as these led them to a deep and continuing distaste for general publicity of any sort about themselves or their Clinic. For years thereafter they flatly refused to give interviews to reporters or writers or allow themselves or the Clinic to be the subject of any nonmedical publication that they could prevent—an attitude which persists just as strongly today at the modern Mayo Clinic as it did in 1910.

Criticism of the Mayo group continued, however, sometimes arising from young doctors who were disgruntled or angry because their applications for training positions at Mayo had been rejected, sometimes from practicing physicians who had lost one too many gall-bladder patients to Will Mayo. And indeed, continuing enmity toward the Mayo brothers on the part of some doctors persists right up to the present day. For example, one criticism that appeared in the early 1900s was the charge of nepotism—that is, the Mayo group were a tight, closed family organization, with family ties and favorable marriages counting more highly than a man's quality and skill in medicine in gaining admission to the group. Such a notion is a little ridiculous today in a group practice which now numbers 650 partners, yet the stories persist. While gathering data for this book in 1978 I encountered a middle-aged physician acquaintance from the West Coast in the lobby of a theater between the acts of a play. When I told him I was working on a book about the Mayo Clinic, he laughed. "You know," he said, "they used to say that the only way a doctor could be appointed to the staff of the Mayo Clinic was to get into, or come out of, a Mayo vagina." And he roared with laughter.

In all fairness, the original charge of nepotism had a kernel of truth to it. Certainly the two brothers ascended to their father's practice in the most natural fashion imaginable—as have many other doctors' sons. Will married a Rochester girl and Charlie married Edith Graham, also of Rochester, while she was serving the Mayos as anesthetist, office nurse, general bookkeeper and secretary. Back in the 1890s Edith's brother Kit, trained in veterinary medicine, went back to earn a medical degree on the strength of the Mayos' invitation to join them. Later Dr. Donald Balfour, coming to the Mayo staff, married Will Mayo's elder daughter, Carrie. The two daughters of Dr. Berkman, an early associate, married Henry Plummer and Starr Judd respectively, and Dr. Stinchfield's daughter Nellie married Dr. William Braash, another early partner. Ultimately Harry Harwick married Kit Graham's daughter Margaret.

All this did indeed seem to be a cozy family arrangement—and it continued as the Clinic staff took shape. Will Mayo had no sons that survived infancy, but Charlie carried on the tradition of Mayo doctors with two sons, Charles William (called "Chuck" to distinguish him from his father) and Joseph. Both went to medical school. Both came back to Rochester for further training, earmarked for partnership on the Mayo Clinic staff when the time came.

Joseph's career was cut short by a tragic accident while he was still in training. During a hunting trip in Wisconsin on a holiday, the Model-A Ford he drove was struck by a train and he was killed. Chuck Mayo, however, carried on the family tradition as a Mayo surgeon and continued active on the staff until his death in 1965, the last of those bearing the Mayo name to be associated with the Clinic up to the present. Chuck's own son, Charles Mayo III, also studied medicine but never fit in comfortably with the Clinic staff and is now in private practice in another city.

Considering the circumstances, it was hardly surprising that such a cozy "family in-group" pattern should have developed. In a tiny town like Rochester in the early 1900s, doctors in the group were naturally and inevitably drawn to one another, and who, precisely, *would* a young doctor in such a place marry if not a nurse who is the sister of a close doctor friend, or a girl who is a daughter of one of the other doctors? Later on the pattern expanded. Doctors on the Clinic staff had sons who studied medicine and, having been raised in the medical atmosphere of Mayo's, those sons quite naturally sought to come back for their specialty training. Ultimately, many ascended to partnership. At present there are literally dozens of second-generation doctors on the Mayo staff and at least one case of a third-generation doctor.

On the other hand, the growth and expansion of the Clinic made ample room for completely unconnected young doctors to come there for training, with the idea that some might later be invited to join the staff. These training recruits, Fellows first in surgery and then in the many medical specialties, came from every state in the Union and from many foreign countries as well. The Mayo group made no bones, in considering applicants for these prized positions, that they were looking for *quality*—bright young physicians with high professional potential. They were picky and often arbitrary in their choices, but once a trainee was chosen, the staff went out of their way to welcome the newcomer and make him feel at home in the Mayo Clinic "family."

One such man was Dr. Heinz Herrmann, today the Chief of Rehabilitation Medicine at a major university hospital rehabilitation center in the South. Now a man in his late fifties and a leader in his field, Herrmann was just twenty-five when he first encountered the Mayo Clinic. Educated in Germany and working as an internist in a hospital in Frankfurt at the end of World War II, with a wife and two small daughters, he was eager to come to America for further specialty training. The procedure was tediously slow in those days. First American friends had to sponsor him, provide travel fare and guarantee his support for a period of five years. Even then it took two years to obtain a visa, and to obtain a visa he had to have a position waiting for him. He wrote to the Mayo Clinic and presented his qualifications. To his amazement, they accepted him as a Fellow in biophysics.

"I will never forget my first introduction to America," Dr. Herrmann told me one evening, relaxing over dinner. "We arrived in New York just before Thanksgiving in nineteen fifty-two and we were practically penniless. Those had been very poor years in Germany since the war, and we had the clothes on our backs and a bag or two and that was about all.

Since we had so little money, we all rode the bus from New York to Rochester, and it was snowing, a bitter cold winter. We arrived in Rochester in the middle of the night with the two kids after this ungodly long bus trip and there was a terrible blizzard outside with this icy wind driving the snow." He laughed. "We felt like Russian refugees arriving in Siberia by cattle car, and my wife was close to tears and the little girls were cold and frightened and wailing."

He sighed. "But they were very good to us there," he said, "very kind, helping us feel at home. There was somebody that met us that night and took us to a furnished apartment the Clinic had found for us to live in, with the rent already paid for the first week and food waiting for us in the refrigerator, the kind of simple kindness that's so important.

"There was a funny story later, too. We were all invited to Thanksgiving dinner by the head of the department I was to be working for, so of course we accepted and went. He happened to have a very large woolly dog, and my daughters, Gertrude and Elsa, who were both very small, were really taken with that dog, which of course was very friendly. Then more guests arrived and things got crowded, so the dog got shooed down to the basement and disappeared. Cocktails were served, and we were introduced, and there was much pleasant conversation, and then when it came time for dinner this enormous turkey was brought in on a platter. It was by all means the most enormous roast fowl those little girls had ever seen in their lives and their eyes goggled with disbelief—and then Elsa, who must have been about four, looked around the room and her eyes widened all the more and finally she tiptoed up to the hostess and pointed to the platter and asked, 'Is that the dog?' The hostess of course reassured her that it was not the dog—it was merely a big turkey—but I don't think she really believed it all through dinner until the large woolly dog finally made a reappearance. Everyone present was vastly amused, and the story became one of those odd Mayo legends that so often are repeated."

Dr. Herrmann's sojourn as a Fellow at Mayo's proved a turning point in his career. After spending a year working in biophysics, a staff man encouraged him to change his professional direction and become a Fellow in physical medicine and rehabilitation, a new medical specialty just beginning to emerge. After his training, Dr. Herrmann moved on to other posts, taking his family with him. Years later his younger daughter, Elsa, went on to medical school and, after taking her M.D., returned to Rochester for postgraduate training in medicine. While she was there, on one occasion, she heard a story told about a little foreign girl and a large woolly dog and a Thanksgiving dinner and she smiled and said, "Yes, I know all about that large woolly dog. I was the little foreign girl who asked the question."

Only one important thing remained unfulfilled in the Mayo brothers' dream for the busy medical institution they had established. Certainly Mayo Clinic had become a broad, comprehensive group practice of medicine and surgery, a purely private practice, but of such high quality it could stand comparison with any other medical institution in the country.

That was the "first leg of the stool" on which everything else depended. The "second leg"—medical research, both in the laboratory and with patients and illnesses—had also evolved at the Clinic, thanks to Dr. Plummer's early urging and in spite of Will Mayo's early misgivings. Research flowered even further after World War I as men and women came to Rochester to devote their full time to this sort of medical pursuit. Early on, interest in this work received a boost from the labors of Dr. Edward C. Kendall and his discovery of thyroxin. Later Kendall turned to isolating hormones from the cortex or outer covering of the adrenal gland. In 1935 he identified a particularly potent cortical hormone called "Compound E," later named cortisone. A Clinic specialist in rheumatic diseases, Dr. Philip S. Hench, discovered that cortisone could have a remarkably beneficial effect in relieving the symptoms of rheumatoid arthritis and other inflammatory diseases. These research discoveries were achievements of such towering significance that Kendall and Hench, together with the Swiss adrenal hormone researcher Tadeus Reichstein, were awarded the Nobel Prize in medicine in 1950.

The "third leg of the stool," however, remained missing at Mayo Clinic: formal, recognized status as a major teaching institution in medicine.

The Mayo brothers were aware of the need as early as 1910. It was not that they weren't training young physicians by then, because they certainly were. In fact, they had some thirty-six Fellows undertaking postgraduate study under their tutelage at the time, mostly in surgery. But there was no *formal* training program. These doctors were learning simply by assisting and observing for varying periods of time. Nor was there any formal professional recognition of their training when they had finished, nor any certification of their advanced qualifications.

In fact, a really sound, organized and comprehensive pattern of graduate medical education simply didn't exist anywhere in the country, and the Mayo brothers wanted to create it in Rochester. What was more, they felt this would be a worthy use for the personal fortune of several million dollars they had built up over the years from fees and astute investments. In truth, this money embarrassed them; they agreed with their father's opinion that it was sinful to be rich and even worse to die rich. As Dr. Will once expressed it, "We are custodians of the sick man's dollar." Both brothers had given long thought to ways that some of their fortune could one day be returned to the people from whom it came, in some fashion related to improvement of the quality of medicine. Devoting it to a permanent, ongoing program of formal graduate medical education in Rochester became a dream for them and finally almost an obsession.

It was needed, beyond doubt. In those days a "specialist" in medicine was anyone who declared himself a specialist. The rich and fortunate doctors went to Europe to study under the great teachers and clinicians of Germany, France and England, and many who stuck with it for three or four years did indeed come home highly qualified to do specialized work. But others claimed the same qualifications after a short summer vacation of study, and no one could tell one from the other.

Then in 1914 the University of Minnesota, which had established a medical school in 1888 and had gradually enlarged and improved it, undertook a vast reorganization of its medical training program and made plans to add a program of graduate work for physicians who had finished medical school and wanted specialist's training—a program of study, hospital work and research that would lead to special advanced degrees. It was the opportunity the Mayos had been looking for. Since there were no better facilities for the advanced study of medicine in all of Minnesota than at the Mayo Clinic in Rochester, it made perfect sense to the brothers that the University of Minnesota and the Mayo Clinic should become affiliated and that they use their surplus money to help develop formal graduate training facilities in Rochester.

The problem was that the Mayo Clinic was not a corporate organization. It was a closely held private practice of medicine, organized as a private partnership, and there was no proper way the tax-supported University of Minnesota could affiliate with such an organization. An ingenious solution was found. On February 8, 1915, the Mayos set up an incorporated Mayo Foundation for Medical Education and Research to control and administer the educational and research phases of their work in Rochester. Trustees of the new foundation were businessmen, including Harry Harwick, rather than the Mayos or any other doctors. Then they transferred an initial gift in excess of $1.5 million into that foundation.

The plan they proposed seemed simple and generous. The Mayo Foundation would be formally and legally linked to the University of Minnesota Medical School. Graduate students, after completion of their basic medical training, would come down to Rochester for additional training in the specialties, with opportunities for formal lectures, hospital experience, study and research. The Mayo Clinic would provide all necessary facilities, and the whole program would be administered by a scientific committee appointed by the foundation. For a trial period—say, five or six years—either the Mayos or the University Regents could withdraw from the arrangement any time they chose. Thereafter, if both agreed, the Mayo endowment would become permanent, with the single stipulation that the endowment income would always be spent on the graduate program in Rochester.

University authorities approved the plan—but an enormous outcry arose from physicians in the area. Twin City doctors who had been hurt by changes in the medical school (many had simply been dismissed from part-time professorships) seized this opportunity to work off their rancor. Other Minnesota doctors who envied or hated the Mayos saw the chance to cut them down to size by attacking the plan. Never before had the brothers been subjected to such vicious public attack on themselves and their organization, to so many slanderous claims and statements against them in newsletters and "fact sheets" that were circulated, or to such diatribes against them and everything they stood for, all under the guise of "protecting the medical school." The Mayos were doing it all for themselves, it was claimed. Their scheme was really an outright grab for control of the medical school. This was no true affiliation, because they would try to control everything; the Mayo Foundation was a phony front that was actually the Mayo Clinic in disguise. The endowment was no gift to the university because all the money would be spent in Rochester anyway and public money as well. In the end the Mayos would be grabbing more patients and fattening their purses. And so on into the night.

In retrospect, it was a singularly disgraceful episode in the history of Minnesota medicine. It must have been a deeply discouraging and painful time for the Mayos as bills were introduced in the Minnesota State Legislature—and passed—forbidding the university authorities from entering into an affiliation with the foundation. The temptation must have been almost irresistible to lash back at their attackers when flat falsehood and bizarre exaggeration were involved, but as Will Mayo once put it, "When you fight with a polecat, you smell like a polecat." The brothers planted their feet and hunched their shoulders and sweated it out, refusing to respond. As recounted earlier, Will Mayo did journey to the Twin Cities to address a legislative committee about the merits of the plan and the unfairness of the opposition's stand, placing himself in the truly grotesque position of using his very considerable oratorical skill to defend himself for offering to give the University of Minnesota a million and a half dollars. There must have been times when both brothers were very nearly ready to quit, throw up their hands and say, "Forget it," but they were stubborn men, and they had not gotten where they were by quitting.

Ultimately, the opposition was overruled and the university affiliation did take place—but only after the Mayo brothers had given in on virtually every point they had originally asked for. The endowment was to be made permanent at once, and both the endowment income and the program of graduate study were to be under complete control of the Board of Regents of the University of Minnesota, not the trustees of the foundation or any scientific committee. The Mayos gave up their right to withdraw during a trial period—only the university could withdraw—and then the idea of a trial period was discarded altogether.

Perhaps the most important of all, there was no stipulation placed upon use of the endowment income, no requirement that *any* of it be spent in Rochester, and few other restrictions except that a small percentage of it was to be devoted to graduate training in medicine abroad, assigned to foreign institutions to further graduate medical studies worldwide. The arrangement finally was voted into effect, and it worked, though hardly in the fashion that the Mayo brothers had hoped might evolve. Medical students did indeed come to Minnesota because they desired the later graduate training in specialties at Rochester. Certainly it was a pioneering advance in the graduate training of physicians in specialized fields of medicine. But after all the bitterness and rancor, there never developed the sense of warmth and close cooperation between the University of Minnesota and the Mayo Clinic, never the sense of mutual trust and understanding, that the Mayos had originally envisioned. The "affiliation" continues to this day, but one still senses a lingering bitterness, a feeling of coolness and wariness between the two institutions. And even today the "affiliation" is more a matter of name than substance. That part of the Mayo dream eluded them to the end—and the university was surely the loser.

The First World War was a watershed for the Mayo Clinic, as it was for virtually every other medical institution in the country. Personnel were scattered far and wide, normal operations were suspended and facilities were turned as needed to military purposes. With the end of the war, however, a new period of growth and expansion began. For the first time a really serious effort was made to recruit Clinic staff in the major medical specialty fields as well as surgery. At the same time a new wave of young doctors came to Rochester for specialty study in these medical fields. Not that surgery was allowed to fade away, however. During the same period, departments of neurosurgery, orthopedic surgery, eye surgery, ear-nose-throat surgery, plastic and reconstructive surgery and rectal surgery were established. Clearly the day of the "general surgeon" who undertook anything and everything known to man was over. Now there were surgeons specializing in the surgery of individual organ systems or even of individual diseases.

This growth brought about the need for more hospital beds and more Clinic facilities. The 1912 addition to St. Mary's Hospital had set aside a fourth floor for medical patients alone. In addition, a small subsidiary hospital across the street from the new Plummer Building, the so-called Colonial Hospital, was intended to serve medical patients as well, except that surgical patients kept crowding them out.

Other things that had previously remained entirely in the Mayo brothers' hands were now institutionalized. For example, the means of handling fees for needy or destitute patients was placed in the hands of a special service department, while the setting and collecting of regular fees was left entirely to the Clinic's business office. Certain old policies the Mayos had established years before were maintained, however. Fees were not standardized as yet but were set in accordance with the patient's ability to pay. Twenty-five percent of the patients paid nothing for their care at the Clinic. Another 30 percent paid the bare cost of their treatment, while the remaining 45 percent paid the rest of the expense of keeping the institution running.

By 1928 a new Clinic building was built, designed by Henry Plummer, fifteen stories tall and still bearing his name. In 1935 a large section was added to the old Colonial Hospital, to be successively enlarged to the present-day 900-bed Rochester Methodist Hospital. In 1937 the first twelve stories of the present-day twenty-story white-and-gray marble monolith of the Mayo Building was dedicated as the Clinic's needs grew.

Meanwhile, some sadder, if inevitable, changes came about. In July 1928 Dr. Will Mayo, then sixty-seven years old and as alert and active as ever, performed his last operation. He decided to quit, as he put it, to make way for younger and surer men. Dr. Charlie Mayo's retirement came a year and a half later under gloomier circumstances: He was quite unexpectedly struck by a retinal hemorrhage in the midst of an operation one morning at a time when his son, Chuck Mayo, was preparing in the next room to assist his father for the first time. He recovered from that blow soon enough but then suffered a succession of debilitating strokes that spelled an end to his active participation in surgery. From that time on the Mayo brothers, individually or together, spent their time traveling, overseeing and advising their partners on Clinic affairs but gradually relinquishing the control they had exercised over the years. On December 31, 1932, both Mayo brothers and Dr. Plummer withdrew from the Board of Governors of the Clinic in favor of three younger men on the staff.

Presently many of the older people, the pioneers, began dying—Henry Plummer, Starr Judd, Maude Mellish Wilson, the Clinic medical editor, and Sister Joseph of St. Mary's Hospital. Then Will Mayo, returning from a winter vacation in Tucson in 1939, began feeling ill and decided to have a checkup at the Clinic. He was found to have cancer of the stomach. He had surgery at once, of course, and seemed to be coming around when he suffered another blow: His brother Charlie, on a shopping trip in Chicago, contracted pneumonia and died on May 26, 1939. Will continued his own recovery for a few weeks but soon relapsed and died on July 28, 1939, just a few days after his seventy-eighth birthday and just over two months after his brother's death.

There were many people who predicted, often with malicious satisfaction, that the Mayo Clinic would shrivel, deteriorate and die after the deaths of the Mayo brothers. "There will be grass growing in the streets of Rochester," one party was quoted as saying. But these doom-singers simply did not take into account the farsightedness, the medical excellence, the moral principles and the great generosity with which the Mayo brothers had endowed the institution they had built. If the Mayo Clinic had been nothing but a private medical practice established for the personal advancement of two clever surgeons, it might well have crumbled and collapsed when the Mayos died. But the Clinic was far more than that. At their deaths it had already become a unique American medical institution, a broad-based and multifaceted center for the treatment of human illness. It was based on principles of private contract and private confidence between doctor and patient, supported by private fees fairly and compassionately set for the services that were rendered, not supported by any tax monies or public funds and free from any government regulations, restrictions, rulings or meddlings. There was no need for the government's thumb in the affairs of the Mayo Clinic and its relationship with its patients. Indeed, it was a showpiece of what private medical practice could accomplish, a tower of excellence in medical care and a world leader in medical progress.

The Mayo Clinic did not wither and die after the death of the Mayo brothers. Far to the contrary, it grew and expanded, broadening its scope, extending its facilities, carrying on its work and caring for an ever-growing volume of patients. Sitting solidly on its three-legged stool of medical

248 / Alan E. Nourse

care, medical research and medical teaching, the Clinic moved steadily forward into modern times. Now, forty years later, it is far larger than when the Mayos died, different in physical appearance as new buildings, new hospitals and new laboratories have been built but unchanged in spirit or purpose since the first partnership was formed in the 1890s.

12

Rochester, Minnesota / *June 1979*

The following Tuesday evening Roger Barton sat in a popular restaurant in Mason City, Iowa, devouring an enormous double-cut pork chop with gusto and watching a fetching young waitress bounce about here and there on her table-waiting duties. She was a new girl here, and when she had come to take his order, Roger could hardly believe his eyes. What was more, when he had later suggested a cruise in his Thunderbird and a drink somewhere after she got off duty, she had not in fact refused out of hand, as was his usual experience. In fact, she had said specifically that she would tell him later and then bounced off to get the salad to go with his pork chop (he had declined baked potato).

Perhaps one reason she had not refused, he reflected, was that he was not sitting here wheezing audibly halfway across the room, dripping, sneezing and constantly blowing his nose, as was also his usual experience. In fact, since his return from Rochester, he had not had a single spell of wheezing—*not one*—and for the first time in his memory he had been enjoying summer evenings with his nose as dry as the Gobi Desert. Indeed, a whole new world of smells and flavors seemed to be opening up for him; his head felt clear, the nagging headache gone, his eyes less puffy than in years. And as a hidden bonus, he was discovering to his amazement that he actually felt *good* most of the time, not half dead and stupefied. He didn't even feel like drinking so much, and although his interest in bosomy young waitresses was every bit as achingly acute as ever, he didn't even miss giving up the baked potato. *Whatever that stuff they gave me up there*, he thought, *it's dynamite, and the blood-pressure medicine isn't so bad either. Hell, even that diet begins to look reasonable, at least parts of it. If I could just get some of this lard off me*—he took another bite of pork chop—*and to think it's taken me all this time to get onto something that really helps! God! If I'd only gone up there ten years ago . . .*

He broke off his reverie when he saw the waitress bouncing back to him with a smile that seemed to be saying *yes— yes—yes*—in perfect rhythm, and he worked his face into his most charming smile.

That same Tuesday evening Giacomo Petri lay resting in his cranked-up bed in his room at St. Mary's Hospital, talking quietly with his wife.

It had been the most harrowing thirty-six hours Mary Petri had ever spent in her life. Jake had gone to surgery the day before, quite early in the morning, and she had seen Dr. O'Shaughnessy for only the briefest moment before he had disappeared into the hospital surgery. "I'll tell you what I can as soon as we're through" was all he would say. "He seems to be in good shape, and that's a plus."

She had waited as the hours passed, pacing the floor, trying to read, staring out the window, mostly watching the minute hand move slowly around the clock on the wall. At one point a nurses' aide had brought her a tray of lunch, a thoughtful gesture except that she couldn't force a bite of it down. Later, desperate to be doing something, anything, she had gone out in the sun and walked the surprisingly short mile down to the Mayo Complex, out among the living, and sat in the little park by the Mayo Building, staring up at Ivan Mestrovic's huge bronze sculpture of Man and Freedom raising its arms in graceful supplication above the north entry. Returning to St. Mary's, she resumed waiting, watching the ever-present wall clock.

And then, at 2:30 in the afternoon, six and one half hours

after Jake had been wheeled away, Dr. Ian O'Shaughnessy reappeared, still dressed in his gray-green scrub suit and cap with a mask dangling around his neck.

He looked excessively tired and suddenly, almost alarmingly, older than Mary had recalled. The humorous sparkle was gone from his eye and a heavy tread seemed to replace his normal bouncing gait. For a moment Mary thought she read disaster in his appearance, but he smiled wearily and shook his head. "Don't worry, it's all right," he said. "These damn things just take it out of a guy my age, that's all. I'm going to have to retire to tonsillectomies."

"Then Jake is okay?" Mary said.

"Jake is fine. He held up like a real fighter, and the procedure went as well as we could possibly ask. We found a good healthy artery in the scalp and took it through the skull and then did the microanastomosis to a branch of the internal carotid above the level of the obstruction."

"A microanastomosis?"

"The artery-to-artery connection," Dr. O'Shaughnessy said. "We made an opening in the carotid artery branch and took the cut end of the scalp artery and then sewed them together into place under a microscope that gave us about twenty diameters magnification. The sutures we used were like pieces of cobweb, so thin you could hardly see them with the naked eye. And then when the connection was made we opened the clamps and let the blood start flowing."

"And the connection went all right?"

The neurosurgeon sighed. "There was an area we weren't really happy with, a little more tension than we liked, so we had to take a couple more stitches than we wanted to. So it wasn't one hundred percent satisfactory from our viewpoint." He laughed. "But then I guess I've never seen one that was, in every way, so maybe that doesn't mean too much. We didn't dare fool with it much more. You have a certain amount of time to work on a thing like this and then everything starts falling apart. I *can* tell you that the extra oxygen going to Jake's brain as soon as that connection was made was already making a significant difference, according to our monitors. And he was already beginning to respond splendidly in the recovery room when I left down there. They'll keep him in the intensive-care unit tonight and get him back to his room tomorrow, if all goes well."

"So now what do I do?" Mary said.

"You keep your fingers crossed. The first twenty-four to thirty-six hours are absolutely critical. If for some reason the new artery connection plugs up with a blood clot, we're right back where we started or worse. If for some reason he should have a stroke involving the right carotid artery or the right side of the brain, he'd be trapped—maybe not trapped quite as badly as if the procedure hadn't been done but trapped just the same, vulnerable to extensive damage or death. If the connection breaks loose, we've lost the ball game. He would simply die of a cerebral hemorrhage." The surgeon looked up at her. "Understand, my dear, I don't think any of these things are going to happen. But they can. Those are the risks we talked about. What I think is going to happen is that he's going to stage an excellent recovery and that you are both going to be on your way home in about a week. I could be wrong, but that's what I think, and it's surely what I hope."

Now, with that critical period fast disappearing behind them, Jake Petri was almost ebullient. "I feel better all over," he said to his wife. "I can't explain it, I just do. I feel stronger. My tongue does what I want it to do. So does my mind. I don't find myself getting confused, stumbling over ideas." They sat and talked, then, and for the first time in months, even turned their thoughts to planning. "Maybe it's time I really did slow down," Jake said. "Just turn the work over to Pete and Harry. Of course, I never saw a lawyer yet who couldn't do better work with a hole in his head—" he pointed to his incision area—"but maybe God is trying to tell me something. And maybe I should listen. Maybe we should take a cruise, a nice long cruise—one of these boat trips to Tahiti. We've got the money. Why not?"

Presently she sensed that he was tiring and got up to leave. "You sleep," she said. "I'll be back in the morning and we can talk some more."

He nodded. "Okay. But before you go, you know something else I noticed? This right hand, the one that was so numb I couldn't hold anything? Well, watch this."

He reached over to the bedside stand with his right hand and picked up a ballpoint pen. Leaning forward in bed so she could see, he held the pen in writing position and slowly raised his right arm out straight. "You see that, Mary? I can hold it just fine now. No numbness. No weakness. No shaking. Already I can hold it just like normal—"

Quite suddenly the pen slid from Jake Petri's grasp and fell clattering to the floor. His right arm gave a couple of convulsive movements and then fell to the bed. Mary heard a gargling sound as Jake tried to speak and then saw him slump back, sagging into the pillow and slumping to one side, his lips and face turning blue.

She rushed to the bed, calling out to him, shaking his shoulder, but there was no response. She screamed and ran into the hall, beckoning as the nurse came running. The nurse sent an aide to call for medical help and then started resuscitation herself, doing many things swiftly and efficiently, all the right things to do, but it was no use after all. It had all been over in the first few seconds.

Giacomo Petri was dead.

Two days later Millie Hulbert had disembarked in Denver from Ozark Airlines Flight 533 from Rochester, feeling weak and wobbly, but determined, and for the first time in her life hired a taxicab to take her from the airport to the Manor. There she was met by a welcoming committee and found a special "Welcome Home, Millie" party scheduled in the common room after dinner that evening. The one or two close friends in whom she had confided her health problem had not, of course, kept the secret too well and the whole Manor was abuzz with the jubilant news: Millie Hulbert had had a breast cancer and had gone to the Mayo Clinic, and they had cured her.

Millie joined the party cheerfully and congratulated all the other people as much as they congratulated her, but in her heart of hearts she harbored no such silly illusions. She had not lived to be eighty-one by virtue of growing stupid.

She knew about breast cancer far too well from the experience of many friends over the years who had succumbed to it, and she did not believe for a minute that she had seen the end of the game.

They had done all she had wanted them to do at Mayo's. There had been more that they could have done, to her misery, which might or might not have helped. But the people there had had the heart and medical judgment and common human decency to allow her to decide to do nothing more. Eighty-one years was a long, rich and full life. She was comfortable and would remain so for two or three more years, maybe more. Then, if recurrence appeared and if push came to shove, there was time enough to do other things. And presently, she felt certain, time would run out and the disease would take her. *But something has to, doesn't it?* she thought. *If not that, then something else—something—who knows?—even worse. Time enough to worry about that when it happens.*

That same Tuesday afternoon in a lawyer's office in Faribault, Minnesota, an angry farmer discussed his problem with his attorney. His wife, never really recovered from her surgery at Mayo's and suffering another acute attack of her colitis, had departed that day for the University Hospital at Iowa City. Her husband had not heard if she had yet arrived. He was preoccupied with making the Mayos pay.

"Oh, we have a splendid case against them," the lawyer said. "Of course, you should understand, it's still highly problematical. I can't imagine they'd ever allow it to go to court. Very bad for the image. Extremely difficult, that sort of thing. No, I think they'll settle out of court."

"What kind of settlement?" the farmer asked suspiciously.

"A good one, we can count on that," the lawyer said. "Nothing of the sort that we're claiming, of course—forget about that. It was only a matter of show. But enough to cover your costs and a little bit more to make you feel better. And *my* fee, of course. A generous settlement—"

That same Tuesday evening Manuela LaBarca was busily stirring about the children's floor of St. Mary's Hospital, playing with her newfound friends, watching the television, coming to life as a child in a fashion that had been impossible in all her nine years of life. She had seen Dr. Norgaard briefly that evening—*"El Animal,"* as she secretly called him—and he had brought her good news. Plans were being made for her transfer by air to the hospital in Mexico City, back to her friends, her home, the people and the language she knew. She would have to come back to Mayo Clinic to be checked in two years. Until then, she would be on her own, building her strength and growing in body and mind. She did not know (but Dr. Norgaard did) that when he saw her next, the small, frail Manuela would be gone forever and the first signs of a strong, healthy, mature and complex young woman would be in her place. And what more, Dr. Norgaard wondered, could one possibly ask?

And what of the future of the Mayo Clinic? One might certainly imagine that it would continue with its work in the future much the same as it has in the past, growing and expanding as demand for its services increased, treating the patients who go there, pursuing its many areas of research and training future young doctors to become experts in their special fields of medicine—in short, serving just as it does today, in a sense, as Medical and Surgical Consultant to the World. To me the idea of serious change in all this was unthinkable. If the Mayo Complex were somehow to vanish from the earth one night by some evil magic, it seemed to me that the loss would be staggering—to patients, to medicine and to the nation.

Yet many that I spoke to in Rochester were very apprehensive. Many considered the prognosis for the Mayo Clinic's future to be extremely guarded. Massive changes in the way medicine would be practiced—in the way "health products would be delivered to the consumer," to borrow the federal medical bureaucrats' favorite language—were already fast appearing on the horizon, and many thought the

Mayo Clinic, as a huge private medical institution, to be especially vulnerable. Everyone I spoke to believed that *some* sort of serious change would be forthcoming there in the future. Some felt the change might be minimal, with the Clinic's basic work continuing much the same as it is today. But others claimed the change would be radical and fundamental, that ultimately the Clinic in anything like its present form was doomed.

I was thinking of this as I sat in the lounge of a West Coast airport waiting for the flight that would take me back to Rochester for the last time before this book was completed. I was mentally reviewing all I had seen and heard at Mayo Clinic in the course of many visits—from doctors, patients, researchers, technicians, cab drivers, townspeople—trying to sort out in my mind just what it was that made Mayo so different from other medical institutions, what they were doing there that really mattered and where the bottom line was from the *patient's* point of view. I found myself returning to a thought I had had one evening much earlier in my Mayo adventure: that really and basically, in medicine of all things, there is just no substitute for quality—and that *this* was the area where Mayo Clinic was most vulnerable of all to future changes in national health-care policy.

I thought about it all through that plane ride back to Minnesota. Certainly, I thought, quality in medical care had to be preserved at all costs as government health programs were developed. I knew that quality existed: I had seen it epitomized, among other places, in a great private medical institution in Rochester, Minnesota. Quality in medical care didn't arise at the Mayo Clinic by accident or by magic. It arose from the vision and labor and real human qualities of a few brilliant men who founded it and of a multitude more who carried on their work.

True, there were holes in the fabric of quality there, sometimes gaping holes—but not very many. The human element—the dedicated concern of one human being for the welfare of another—tended to get lost in the sheer *machinery* of medicine there, but the human element was present all the same, however elusive it sometimes seemed when you tried to pin it down. Maybe the human element in medicine is always hard to pin down—but it has been present for thousands of years. Mayo's only carries on an ancient tradition.

One thing was certain, I thought, as the plane homed in on Minneapolis airport: Quality in medicine has always been an absolute. You can't have "a little quality" in this area, any more than a woman can be somewhat pregnant, or a surgical pack almost sterile. It's got to be all or nothing; when a person's health and life are in the balance, who wants to settle for "a little quality"?

So what about the threat to quality at Mayo? Back in Rochester, I raised the question of the Mayo Clinic's future with Art Amundson in his office high on the eleventh floor of the Mayo Building. Art rumpled his iron-gray hair and grimaced with his Boris Karloff face and spread his hands in a gesture of helplessness. "Who knows?" he said. "We try to look ahead, and you'd better believe that we worry. Obviously, if we're allowed to, we want to go right on doing what we've always done, treating the patients that come to us, building and enlarging our facilities as we need to, aiming for the quality of medicine that we've always aimed for. But we may not be allowed to do that. There's no question that government controls and rules and regulations are looming up in the future, and nobody can guess what may happen." He stared unhappily out at the summer sky.

"But how can government controls seriously alter a medical institution like Mayo's?" I asked. "What can they actually *do*?"

"They can do lots of things to Mayo's if they choose to," Art said. "For example: If they were to institute too rigid, too arbitrary cost controls on the diagnostic procedures we do here, they could very quickly destroy the fantastic diagnostic capability we've spent over seventy years developing here— and cripple the quality of medicine we could practice. If our doctors had to write three-page justifications for every X ray they wanted to take, every blood study they wanted to order, every biopsy they wanted to perform, they would have no time left to see patients—a self-limiting problem, of course. If a rigidly cost-conscious Department of Health, Education and Welfare were suddenly to block the development of any further high-cost medical technology, they could kill projects like our Dynamic Spatial Reconstructor dead as a dodo bird—and then there just wouldn't *be* any. Worse yet, suppose a national health-insurance program were adopted that designated Mayo Clinic exclusively as a regional medical center to serve a couple of neighboring states and nothing more. Well, consider for a minute what that would mean. Everything we're able to do here depends on a vast patient base, two hundred and seventy-five thousand patients a year and still going up. That's the base that keeps our six hundred and eighty staff doctors—some of the finest specialists in the world—busy. That's the base that allows us to train six hundred or seven hundred young doctors every year. That's the base that allows us to maintain our vast research program and to provide quality medical care for each of those patients. But if we were suddenly cut down to a mere regional institution serving just Minnesota, Wisconsin and Iowa, for example, with a patient base cut down to twenty-five thousand patients a year, it would kill us. The once great Mayo Clinic would become just one more small, mediocre regional medical center. With our patient base gone, the staff would go. The research would die. The teaching would die. The quality of medicine would die."

For the first time since I had met him, Art Amundson looked tired and gray and discouraged. "The ironic part of it," he said, "is that government rules and controls could never have *created* the Mayo Clinic. There is no way they could have come close. It was created by medical skill and ingenuity and human concern and private enterprise, and it needs liberal quantities of all those things to survive in the future. Fortunately, there may be a way that we *can* survive. One thing we've been fighting for is the idea of preserving places like this as special National Health Resources under whatever government health program is finally enacted. In addition to Mayo's this would include places like the Cleveland Clinic, the Ochsner Clinic in New Orleans, the Ford Clinic in Detroit, Leahy in Boston and others of the sort all over the country. It would allow them to draw patients from the whole nation wide and to carry on the big, massive teaching and research programs they already have with a minimum of interference. These are the places where progress in medicine is going to come from, where quality can be preserved at its best. We think it may work, and Congress is definitely interested—so for now we're pretending it's going to happen, proceeding with our plans for continuing growth and expansion and improvement of our services. But we really don't know."

Later, as I walked around the town of Rochester and saw the ambulances turning in at Rochester Methodist Hospital, saw the doctors hurrying across the street from the Mayo Building, saw the students and their wives gathering for celebration dinners after the close of medical school, saw the multitude of small quiet homes in that small quiet Midwest city housing the staff and Fellows of the Mayo Clinic, I could not believe that anything disastrous was really going to happen here. I did not see any grass growing in the streets of Rochester. Here was an American landmark of medicine, serving the nation, quietly going about its business proving that the private practice of medicine could provide the best that was available anywhere. What was started many decades ago by an irascible old man and his two brilliant sons still stands as a monument to what determination and excellence can do.

And in Rochester that night a graduate of the Mayo Medical School was making plans to go elsewhere for his graduate training. At the same time an airplane landing from Minneapolis was discharging a young man trained in an Eastern medical school and now arriving in Rochester to begin his specialty training. A thousand patients were gathering to be seen by Mayo Clinic doctors the next day, and someone in a laboratory in the Medical Sciences Building was finally closing in on the ultimate answer to a problem that might, in the fullness of time, save 100,000 lives. A cardiac surgeon was rejoicing in his heart over the salvation of one sick young patient, and a neurosurgeon was grieving in his heart at the loss of one sick elderly patient, and elsewhere in Rochester the quiet, complex machinery of good medical care moved on.

Afterword

Roger Barton's total costs for his five-day examination at the Mayo Clinic amounted to $723.43. Without asking, he was offered the option of paying this bill in three equal monthly installments. He accepted the offer with alacrity.

Millie Jordan Hulbert's total billings for her care in Rochester, including all Mayo Clinic services, surgeons' fees, operating-room costs and twelve days' hospitalization, came to $3,540.00. Medicare paid in full for all but two items, which they disallowed: $11.85 for medications she took home with her and 40 cents for a milkshake she had requested one very hot afternoon. Millie felt, with no little disdain, that they might have allowed the milkshake, considering the size of the federal Medicare budget.

Manuela LaBarca's bill, after her difficult surgery and her stormy postoperative hospital course, reached a total of $13,461.23. This was paid in full by her father at the time of her transfer to Mexico City, by a check drawn on the Banco de Oaxaca. Six months later the Mayo Clinic received an additional check in the amount of $50,000 in Manuela's name as a gift to further their work in treating congenital heart disease.

Mary Petri, wife and widow of Giacomo Petri, received a bill in the amount of $5,420.35 covering her husband's hospital costs, Clinic costs, operating-room costs and surgery. Accompanying the bill was a letter from Dr. Ian O'Shaughnessy expressing his personal distress at the outcome of Jake's illness and detailing briefly the findings at autopsy: a sudden, massive hemorrhage from the carotid artery branch above the site of the bypass—a hazard that no one could have foreseen but that always could occur in a situation of that sort.

The bill for my own examination at the Mayo Clinic, involving about four days, was $766.70. I was not, however, allowed to pay a penny, since the Mayo Clinic to this day will not accept a fee from a physician or his immediate dependent family.

Sarah Swedman's husband's litigation was, as predicted, settled out of court. No one but the Swedmans' lawyer was happy with the result.